Beating Ankylosing Spondylitis Naturally

By Dr. Scott A. Johnson

COPYRIGHT 2014 Scott A. Johnson

All Rights Reserved. No part of this publication may be reproduced or transmitted in any form or by any means, electronic or mechanical, including photocopying and recording, or introduced into any information storage and retrieval system without the written permission of the copyright owner. Brief quotations may be used in reviews with proper citation.

Beating Ankylosing Spondylitis Naturally/Scott A. Johnson

ISBN-13: 978-1502403759

ISBN-10: 1502403757

Discover more books by Scott A. Johnson at authorscott.com

Published by
Scott A. Johnson Professional Writing Services, LLC

Printed by CreateSpace, an Amazon.com Company

Cover design: Scott A. Johnson, Copyright © 2014 Scott A. Johnson

Cover image credit: Sebastian Kaulitzki/Shutterstock

DISCLAIMERS OF WARRANTY AND LIMITATION OF LIABILITY

The author provides all information on an "as is" and "as available" basis. Author makes no representations or warranties of any kind, expressed or implied, as to the information, materials, or products mentioned.

Always consult a qualified medical professional before using any dietary supplement or natural product and seek the advice of your physician with any questions you may have regarding any medical condition. The information contained in this book is for educational and informational purposes only, and it is not meant to replace medical advice, diagnosis, or treatment in any manner. Never delay or disregard professional medical advice. Use the information solely at your own risk; the author accepts no responsibility for the use thereof.

The Food and Drug Administration (FDA) has not evaluated the statements contained in this book. The information and materials are not meant to diagnose, prescribe, or treat any disease, condition, illness, or injury.

Table of Contents

Foreword	7
Introduction	8
What is Ankylosing Spondylitis?	11
The Breakdowns in Standard Treatment Options	20
Eating and Ankylosing Spondylitis	29
Physical Activity and Ankylosing Spondylitis	39
Natural Remedies for Ankylosing Spondylitis	57
Lifestyle Considerations and Ankylosing Spondylitis	96
Conclusion	104
References	108

Foreword

Much praise for Beating Ankylosing Spondylitis Naturally !!!

I have been a chiropractor for 17 years and I have utilized every form of physical medicine and even supplementation to compliment my practice.

I can honestly say that I have always found cases of ankylosing spondylitis extremely difficult to treat effectively, if at all. In this book Dr. Scott Johnson does an outstanding job of outlining not only what the general public and patients need to know and do to effectively treat this disease, but he gives the practitioner the tools to assist them.

His writing style is second to none when it comes to educational and informational books regarding natural approaches to almost any disease process and this book is no exception.

I am excited at the prospect of not only utilizing this book in my practice but to share it with colleagues. If you or someone you know suffers from ankylosing spondylitis or if you are treating patients with this disease this book is a must read and necessary resource. I highly recommend it.

Dr. George Hoogeveen, D.C.

Introduction

This book is intended to share my personal experience with ankylosing spondylitis (AS) and to help both patients and healthcare practitioners learn how to incorporate natural methods to manage the disease. I share it out of desire that others will benefit from what I have learned over nearly a decade of managing the disease and its many symptoms. I share it to provide hope to those who may feel none and ease suffering. I am frequently asked how I manage this debilitating disease naturally and this book will now make the information widely available to any who desire to learn what I do.

I was officially diagnosed with ankylosing spondylitis in 2005, though my journey with it started long before this. I suspected that I had AS for approximately three years before I went to the doctor to get the official diagnosis. How did I know this? I have a family member who also endures AS, who was diagnosed at a much younger age than me because his AS had progressed more rapidly. After years of being told that his back pain was just growing pains (his pain started in his early teens), a knowledgeable physician with familiarity with AS (because he too has it) explained that he had an inflammatory disease that causes the vertebrae in the spine to fuse together. This fusion causes pain, inflammation and reduced spinal mobility.

Healthy spine   Ankylosing spondylitis

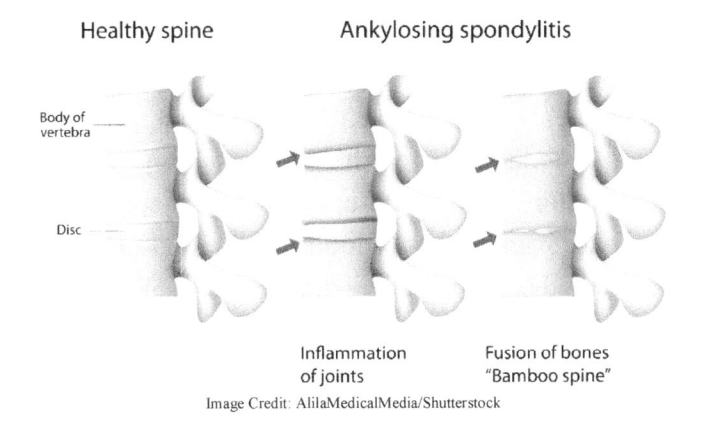

Body of vertebra

Disc

Inflammation of joints   Fusion of bones "Bamboo spine"

Image Credit: AlilaMedicalMedia/Shutterstock

When I began to experience severe back pain and stiffness upon waking in the morning—sometimes so bad my back would lock up and I would have to crawl out of bed—I was already familiar with my family member's diagnosis and the customary disease symptoms. I was in my mid-20s, married with children, and with my whole life ahead of me. I was largely in denial that I had this disease, because I had witnessed others who had AS—now in their 50s—with completely fused spinal columns, making it necessary for them to walk with a cane, and left them without the ability to turn their heads without turning their whole body. In addition, I had recently seen an obituary in the local newspaper that attributed the death of a male in his 30s to complications of AS. I somehow thought that if I didn't get officially diagnosed, I wouldn't experience the symptoms, nor the progression, of the disease.

After a few years of some good mornings and an increasing number of bad mornings with lots of pain in my lower back, I finally decided to go to the doctor. Knowing the difficulty my brother had in getting an accurate diagnosis, I made an appointment with the same physician that diagnosed his condition years before. After describing my symptoms, a physical examination, blood work, and x-rays, I received the anticipated diagnosis of ankylosing spondylitis.

I experienced the typical rush of emotions—as did my family—about what this meant for my future. Was I condemned to a life of pain, stiffness, and reduced functionality? Would this affect my ability to support my family? Would it shorten my lifespan so that I would miss important events in my children's lives? How much would treatment and medications cost over my lifetime? After this initial distress, I determined to keep a positive attitude and manage the condition as best I could by becoming a master of it.

What is ankylosing spondylitis?

AS is a mysterious disease that few have ever heard of and even fewer can pronounce correctly. AS is a progressive arthritic condition that primarily affects the spine. It causes inflammation of the spine and/or adjacent structures of the vertebrae, leading to severe, chronic pain and stiffness. The discomfort is worst after periods of rest, and may improve with movement and heat. Discomfort may start on one side of the lower back or both sides, gradually becoming persistent and spreading up the spine, into the neck, and often radiating through the buttocks and down the legs.

Ankylosing spondylitis was long believed to be an autoimmune disorder; however, because its mechanism of development and progression involves the innate immune system it is truly an autoinflammatory condition.[1] This relatively new distinction of illnesses causes systemic inflammation due to dysfunction of the innate immune system. The innate immune system is the division of the immune system present at birth and the body's first line of defense against germs. It consists of cells and proteins always present and (monocytes, natural killer cells, basophils, eosinophils, neutrophils) prepared to fight a limited number of invading pathogens.

The innate immune system activates the cells mentioned above in response to invading pathogens, which secrete cytokines that trigger inflammation. In autoinflammatory conditions the innate immune system triggers this process without an actual attack from invading pathogens.

Conversely, autoimmune disorders involve the adaptive—or humoral—immune system, which comprises specialized and sophisticated cells that respond as a second line of defense when the innate immune system is unable to neutralize invading pathogens. The adaptive immune system produces antibodies in response to antigens that results in the destruction and removal of the harmful pathogens.

When an autoimmune disorder occurs, the immune system goes awry and does not properly distinguish between healthy tissues and antigens. This dysfunction results in the destruction of normal, healthy tissues and elevated inflammation.

The sooner the diagnosis, the better the prognosis for AS patients, as early detection allows for better management of the diseases before its symptoms begin to cascade.[2] The same is true for incorporating natural remedies, the sooner you start using them the more likely you are to experience results. Diagnosis involves the following:
- *Physical Exam* – spine, pelvis, sacroiliac joints, heels, chest, ability to bend in different directions, and chest expansion capability.

- *Medical History* – duration and specific location of pain, whether pain improves or is worse with movement, if pain and stiffness is more intense first thing in the morning, family history of back problems or arthritis, and the presence of other health conditions (skin rashes, eye problems, fatigue, gastrointestinal disorders).
- *Radiologic Imagery* – X-ray or magnetic resonance imagery (MRI) to check for changes in the spine or sacroiliac joints consistent with AS.
- *Laboratory Tests* – a blood test to check for the presence of the HLA-B27 gene.

Clinical observations suggest that women experience AS differently than men, with symptoms frequently starting in the neck rather than the back. Women can be more difficult to diagnose properly because spinal radiographic changes—those visible through electromagnetic radiation imagery—and standard indications of AS, are generally less visible in women. In addition, women tend to have a higher disease burden, greater incidence of peripheral arthritis, and are less responsive to treatment [3,4]

AS belongs to a group of diseases known as seronegative spondyloarthropathies, which also includes reactive arthritis (Reiter's syndrome), inflammatory bowel disease related arthritis, and psoriatic arthritis. This group of conditions is generally negative for rheumatoid factor (RF), distinguishing it from rheumatoid arthritis, but shares common factors such as uveitis, oral ulcers, rash, and inflammation of the tendon and ligament insertion sites (enthesitis).

Because AS is progressive, it can affect virtually any joint in the body (jaw, shoulders, knees, ribs, hips, wrist, fingers, heel, toes, etc.). In addition it can cause a variety of other health conditions including cervical myelopathy—compression of the cervical spinal cord leading to interrupted nerve signal transmission, fatigue due to decreased production of red blood cells, uveitis in about one-third of patients, psoriasis, bowel dysfunction or lesions, bladder and sexual dysfunction (especially if nerves at the base of the spine are damaged or scarred). Rarely the lungs (scarring or fibrosis at the top of the lungs, breathing impairment due to chest wall restriction, sleep apnea, abnormal accumulation of air in the space between the lungs and chest cavity, called pneumothorax) and heart (enlargement or dysfunction of the aorta, cardiomyopathy, reduced blood supply to the heart, myocarditis—inflammation of the heart muscle leading to conduction disturbances) may be affected.[5,6]

It is a uncommon disease that is estimated to affect about 129 Caucasians out of 100,000 in the United States[7]—or just over one-tenth of a percent of the population. It is estimated to be even rarer among some ethnicities, including African Americans.[8] Men are more likely to develop AS than women, though the gender gap in diagnoses appears to be shrinking. AS is most frequently diagnosed from adolescence through age 30, though it may be diagnosed later in adulthood due to its slow progression and diagnosis difficulties.

There is no known definitive cause or cure for AS currently, but scientists have discovered that individuals who possess the human leukocyte antigen B27 (HLA-B27) gene are more susceptible to it. Of those who have been diagnosed with AS, approximately 28 to 44 percent possess the gene, with some countries—like the United Kingdom—approaching 95 percent of patients possessing the gene.[9] Physicians will often perform a blood test to determine the presence of the HLA-B27 gene to guide his or her diagnosis. However, it is important to remember that not all people who have the HLA-B27 gene develop AS, nor does everyone who has AS have the gene.

The HLA-B family of genes is responsible for helping the immune system distinguish normal body tissues from foreign invaders (viruses and bacteria). Although the connection between HLA-B27 and AS is still poorly understood, it is possible that alterations in the gene cause the immune system to attack its own body tissues. It is estimated that less than 10 percent of the world population possesses the HLA-B27 gene and the majority who do have it do not have AS.[10]

Another gene associated with AS is the endoplasmic reticulum aminopeptidase 1 (ERAP1) polymorphism.[11,12,13,14] ERAP1 provides instruction for making the protein that is active in the endoplasmic reticulum (ER)—a network of tubules and sacs in the cell that manufacture membranes, secretory proteins, hormones, and antibodies (rough ER). The ER also produces enzymes that aid detoxification, aid muscle contraction, synthesize male and female hormones and is involved in carbohydrate and lipid synthesis (smooth ER).

A dysfunction of ERAP1 affects the immune system's response in a significant manner. First, ERAP1 is involved in mediating cytokine response, which affects the normal inflammatory response. If ERAP1 is not working correctly, excess inflammation can occur. Second, ERAP1 is responsible for displaying protein peptides from within the cell to the immune system so immune cells can detect whether the peptide is normally found within the body or foreign (viral or bacterial pathogens). If the body is unable to detect foreign pathogens because of alteration in the ERAP1 gene, its ability to fight infection is diminished. Scientists believe that interactions with HLA-B27 and ERAP1 may play an important role in AS pathogenesis.

Other genes that have been linked to AS include the IL1A and IL23R genes. IL1A is involved in the production of the proinflammatory protein interleukin-1 alpha, which is involved in the inflammatory response, helps protect the body from foreign invaders, and aids the bone resorption process—the breakdown and removal of old bone tissue. Alteration in this gene likely causes increased inflammation.

IL23R is also involved in immune system function by producing interleukin 23 receptor—a protein found in immune system cell membranes that helps coordinate the immune system's response to pathogens and triggers inflammation. Because it is involved in the immune responses to both pathogens and inflammation, alteration of IL23R may encourage excess inflammation and improper responses by the immune system to normal body tissues. IL23R is also influential in the gut inflammatory response, which may increase the risk of inflammatory bowel diseases.

Other scientists have investigated—and are still investigating—a link between pathogenic bacteria and initiation of AS, though the evidence remains inconclusive.[15] Some studies have linked the initiation and progression of inflammatory activity and AS with the pathogen *Klebsiella pneumoniae*[16,17,18] a gram-negative bacteria that can cause pneumonia, bloodstream infections, wound or surgical site infections, and meningitis. Other pathogenic bacteria that are more prevalent in patients with AS, or have been linked to exacerbation of symptoms or triggering AS include staphylococci,[19] *Escherichia coli*,[20] and *Chlamydia pneumoniae*.[21] Some research even suggests that the HLA-B27 gene predisposes AS patients to an altered gut bacteria environment that favors disease.[22]

This pathogenic bacteria connection to AS involves the theory of molecular mimicry. The theory is that tissues and cells normally found within the human body share similarities—structural, functional, or immunological—with pathogens. Because of these shared similarities the body's immune system erroneously identifies normal cells and tissues—that resemble pathogens—as harmful and mount an attack to neutralize them and remove them from the body, as if they were harmful pathogens.[23,24] In other words, the immune system is somewhat tricked into attacking normal cells and tissues by bacteria that share similar characteristics.

Another theory related to molecular mimicry suggests that pathogens can persist in the human body in a dormant state through specific survival mechanisms. Researchers hypothesize that pathogenic organisms endure within the spine and other tissues in an inactive sate by employing protective mechanisms that keep them alive, but temporarily reduce their ability to replicate and spread. These pathogens can then become reactivated by an external or internal trigger to cause disease initiation and progression.[25,26]

This theory appears to have some credence with spondyloarthritis, where researchers propose that bacteria persist in the spine or related tissues.[27] These pathogens must be reactivated somehow to make them susceptible to antimicrobial agents and remove the possible cause and progression of disease. It has also been suggested that the HLA-B27 gene misfolds proteins—decreasing detection of pathogenic bacteria by the immune system and increasing inflammatory pathways—allowing migration of infected cells to membranes and tissues prone to spondyloarthritis.[28] Therefore, pathogens remain dormant and hidden in tissues until reactivated. These theories are not definitive, but based on the growing body of evidence connecting pathogens, the HLA-B27 gene, and AS they are quite plausible.

While heredity is a factor—HLA-B27, IL1A, and IL23R genes and a family history of AS—genetic factors do not doom you to getting AS. In fact, the chances that you will pass the HLA-B27 gene to your children is small and the chance that your children will have AS is even smaller. Even among family members who have AS, disease progression and symptoms can be significantly different. It is more probable that lifestyle and environmental factors are required to trigger the onset of AS.

The Breakdowns in Standard Treatment Options

Disease progression varies widely among AS patients, with some people experiencing periods of remission, and others continually in chronic and severe pain. There is no known cure for ankylosing spondylitis currently and so physicians and other healthcare practitioners strive to relieve symptoms and control disease progression as much as possible. This is accomplished largely through medications such as non-steroidal anti-inflammatory drugs (NSAIDs), muscle relaxers, pharmaceutical analgesics (pain relieving medications), corticosteroids, disease-modifying antirheumatic drugs (DMARDs), and biologic agents.

NSAIDs are usually the physician's first line of defense against the pain and inflammation associated with AS. This has been the cornerstone of treatment during the early phases of AS for decades. NSAIDs help relieve pain by blocking cyclooxygenase (COX) enzymes that the body uses to create prostaglandins—hormone-like lipids that control inflammation and blood flow in response to irritation, injury, tissue damage, and infection—and inhibiting arachidonic acid synthesis. The synthesis of arachidonic acid significantly increases inflammation. Most NSAIDs—with the exception of celcoxib—control inflammation by blocking the COX-1 and COX-2 enzymes. Arachidonic acid is converted to prostaglandins by the COX enzymes causing an inflammatory response.

The COX-1 enzyme is normally found throughout the body and helps create prostaglandins involved in key bodily functions like stomach mucous lining production, regulation of gastric acid, platelet formation for blood clotting, and kidney water excretion. The COX-2 enzyme is triggered by an immune response (irritation, illness, injury, etc.) and is more involved in the inflammatory response, signaling pain and inflammation.

Because the COX-1 enzyme is responsible for important housekeeping functions, it is disadvantageous to block its action. On the other hand it is desirable to selectively inhibit the activity of the COX-2 enzyme in efforts to control inflammation, pain, swelling, and redness. One of the most common side effects experienced with a traditional NSAID (blocks both COX-1 and COX-2 enzymes) is stomach discomfort or ulcers. Why? Because the COX-1 enzyme can't perform its function of producing prostaglandins that generate the protective inner lining of the stomach. Unable to perform this duty efficiently, stomach ulcers and irritation frequently occur.

Another serious side effect of long-term NSAID usage is kidney failure and liver damage. These medications are estimated to cause liver damage in less than one percent of people who take them, but a cumulative effect may occur with concurrent alcohol use.[29] NSAIDs reduce creatinine—a byproduct of creatine muscle metabolism—clearance, which is a good indicator of kidney function. If excess creatinine is found in the blood, this suggests that the kidneys are not effectively filtering small molecules out of the blood. Chronic use of NSAIDs can lead to kidney disease (chronic interstitial nephritis—inflammation of the spaces between the kidney tubules) and kidney failure in rare cases.[30,31] Depending on the specific NSAID, there is a long list of additional side effects associated with their use, such as nausea, vomiting, diarrhea, constipation, rash, dizziness, headache, and edema. The longer an NSAID is used the more likely side effects will occur, and since AS patients must continually take something to reduce inflammation and pain, adverse effects are almost expected.

Knowing the serious and frequent kidney and stomach problems linked to NSAIDs that inhibit both COX enzymes, pharmaceutical companies set out to create a new drug that selectively inhibits only the COX-2 enzyme. Unfortunately, while this was a noble endeavor, the pharmaceutical companies traded kidney and stomach side effects for increased cardiovascular risks.[32] The increased risk of cardiovascular events like stroke and heart attack became such a concern that two of the major

COX-2 inhibiting NSAIDs, Vioxx® and Bextra® were both removed from the market, many other drugs in development were withdrawn or not approved for use by the FDA, and the one remaining on the market (Celebrex®) must carry the sternest "black box" warning.

> **WARNING: CARDIOVASCULAR AND GASTROINTESTINAL RISKS**
> *See full prescribing information for complete boxed warning*
>
> **Cardiovascular Risk**
> - CELEBREX, may cause an increased risk of serious cardiovascular thrombotic events, myocardial infarction, and stroke, which can be fatal. All NSAIDs may have similar risks. This risk may increase with duration of use. Patients with cardiovascular disease or risk factors for cardiovascular disease may be at greater risk. *(5.1, 14.7)*
> - CELEBREX is contraindicated for the treatment of peri-operative pain in the setting of coronary artery bypass graft (CABG) surgery. *(4, 5.1)*
>
> **Gastrointestinal Risk**
> - NSAIDs, including CELEBREX, cause an increased risk of serious gastrointestinal adverse events including bleeding, ulceration, and perforation of the stomach or intestines, which can be fatal. These events can occur at any time during use and without warning symptoms. Elderly patients are at greater risk for serious gastrointestinal (GI) events. *(5.4)*

Source: U.S. Food and Drug Administration. Highlights of prescribing information. Celebrex® (celecoxib) capsules. Accessed September 8, 2014 from http://www.accessdata.fda.gov/drugsatfda_docs/label/2008/020998s027lbl.pdf.

Muscle relaxers may be prescribed in conjunction with NSAIDs or analgesics to help control muscle related pain and spasms. When your joints are inflamed and painful, surrounding muscles are frequently affected and some may experience spams upon lying down, as your muscles adapt to being able to relax after being tensed in response to the joint pain. Muscle relaxers work by depressing the central nervous system, frequently causing drowsiness, which can be very problematic when working, operating equipment, or driving. It is not recommended to drive if you take a muscle relaxer because of this effect. In addition, muscle relaxers may cause addiction, dizziness, urinary retention, fatigue, headache, and dry mouth.

Analgesics may be given alone or in combination with NSAIDs. Acetaminophen, or aspirin, is not an NSAID but a pain reliever (analgesic) that is strongly associated with acute liver failure. In fact, acetaminophen is currently the leading cause of acute liver failure in both the United States and the United Kingdom.[33,34] Other side effects of acetaminophen include duodenal ulcers, abdominal pain, nausea, stomach inflammation, liver toxicity, black stools, bleeding on the brain, and dizziness.

A physician will often prescribe the lowest dose of milder NSAIDs first for AS patients in efforts to reduce the risk of side effects. However, this dosage and/or the specific medication often need to be changed to maintain relief from pain and inflammation.

If NSAIDs do not control the pain sufficiently, corticosteroid injections are usually the next step. Corticosteroids are a class of medications related to steroids, similar to the cortisone naturally produced by the body, and can be injected directly into the site of pain to reduce inflammation. If the injection is successful and makes it to the intended place within the body, corticosteroids can provide inflammation relief for months and even years. The most common side effects include pain and swelling at the injection site, stomach discomfort, rapid heartbeat, nausea, vomiting, sleep disturbance, diminished wound healing, acne, and a metallic taste in the mouth.

Other less common, but more serious side effects include vision problems, rapid weight gain, mood disorders, pancreatitis, extremely high blood pressure, death of nearby bone, nerve damage, and low potassium. In addition, corticosteroids may suppress immune system activity—inhibiting white blood cell activity—making you more susceptible to infections. Clinical observations suggest that repetitive cortisone injections cause cumulative tissue (cartilage and tendons) and bone damage, making it very important to limit the number of injections received during your lifetime.

A relatively new class of drugs, conventional disease-modifying antirheumatic drugs (DMARDs) work differently than other medications used for AS. They work to slow down progressive joint destruction, associated organ damage, and suppress the immune response. The most common DMARDs used for AS are methotrexate and sulfasalazine. These medications are generally used for those who either do not respond or build a tolerance to standard NSAID treatment. They are slow acting and may take weeks or months to provide noticeable relief. DMARDs decrease blood cell production and increase your risk of infections. In addition, other side effects include sore throat, fever, jaundice, unexplained bruising or bleeding, increased photosensitivity, decreased sperm count, and liver damage (methotrexate—when taken for long periods of time).

Biologic therapies (or biologics), are given to patients who do not respond to conventional DMARDs and have to be administered by injection or intravenous infusion. As of 2014, four biologics have been approved by the U.S. Food and Drug Administration for the treatment of AS—adalimumab, etanercept, golimumab, and infliximab. These four biologics decrease inflammation and alter disease effect on the body by suppressing tumor necrosis factor (TNF-α)—a cytokine involved in the inflammatory response. In a healthy person, TNF-α is controlled naturally; however, in a person with AS, higher levels of TNF-α are not controlled adequately leading to excess inflammation and joint damage. Biologics reduce your ability to fight infections and increase the risk of developing a serious infection. Besides the typical redness, irritation and swelling at the injection site, biologics may also cause headache, nausea, back pain (seems counterintuitive), numbness, chest pain, vision problems, shortness of breath, seizures, rash or hives, joint pain in a different location, unusual bleeding, and dizziness.

In severe cases of AS, surgery may be necessary, though it is rare and should only be used in extreme cases. If the spine is fused in a severely stooped position making it impossible to stand erect, surgery to correct this curvature is sometimes recommended. This is performed by cutting through the spine so that it can be realigned to a more vertical position and then inserting metal hardware to maintain this position of the spine. Additionally, if joints (hips or knees) are worn out, joint replacement surgery may be necessary. Neither of these surgeries are easy or risk free. In fact, the spinal surgery is considered high risk and should only be performed by a surgeon with significant experience in the procedure. Surgery doesn't work for everyone, so it should be performed only as a very last resort.

Given the conventional treatment options and their associated risks, things may seem bleak for patients with AS. However, I can tell you from personal experience that with the right lifestyle modifications and help from some natural remedies, relief is possible. I am now almost a decade free of using any drugs—even over the counter drugs—to manage my AS.

My personal experience is that I was initially prescribed a low dose of indomethacin by my family physician, which seemed to reduce the pain rather well at first. I took this while I waited to see a rheumatologist, who validated this action as a reasonable first step to manage the pain I was experiencing. However, the lower dose quickly stopped providing complete relief and I was advised by the rheumatologist to increase the dosage that I was taking. I was also offered the choice of taking celecoxib, but after reading the warning label on the box I decided against taking it.

Not long after increasing the indomethacin dose, I began having severe stomach pain, which turned out to be an ulcer from the indomethacin. My rheumatologist then prescribed a proton-pump inhibitor (PPI) to reduce the stomach pain. Proton-pump inhibitors work by blocking the enzyme responsible for producing stomach acid, which then allows ulcers to heal in a less acidic environment. Unfortunately, the PPI only provided relief for about two weeks before the stomach pain returned. At this point I felt that I needed to choose between back pain or stomach pain, so I stopped taking the indomethacin in hopes that my ulcer would quickly heal.

During this frustrating period, I began doing my own research to find answers to my health conditions without the use of side effect prone medications. Through painstaking research and lots of prayer, I found an herbal remedy that healed my stomach ulcer and restored my gastrointestinal health. I also found a collection of dietary supplements that provided relief from the back pain (more to come on these later).

Eating and Ankylosing Spondylitis

Eating is the foundation of your health and you must treat it as such. You can't put garbage in your body and expect anything but garbage results for your health. The intent of this book is not to have a broad and all-inclusive discussion about proper nutrition. I feel I have discussed these adequately in my other books and invite you to read them for more in-depth information on what it means to eat better. For this text I will focus on eating and how it specifically relates to AS.

The foods you eat can either increase or reduce inflammation. Understanding how food affects your inflammation is important in maintaining a normal inflammatory response and reducing the pain associated with increased inflammation. It may be wise to keep a food journal to monitor how certain foods affect your pain level and the way you feel. Some foods, herbs, and spices that may help reduce inflammation include:

- Dark chocolate (at least 70% cacao) – Scientists have recently discovered that friendly bacteria living in the gut like *Bifidobacterium* and lactic acid bacteria—devour and ferment dark chocolate, producing anti-inflammatory compounds.[35] Eating dark chocolate regularly is also associated with a decrease in serum C-reactive protein (CRP) levels.[36] CRP levels are checked to determine inflammation levels in the body. Levels rise during AS flare-ups and when inflammation is systemic—throughout the body.

- Oily fish – Your body uses omega-3 fatty acids found in oily fish—like salmon and mackerel—to create bioactive lipid compounds called resolvins and protectins.[37,38] After being produced by the body, resolvins and protectins help maintain a normal inflammatory response in different ways.[39] Resolvins are produced by EPA and interact with the portion of your immune system that resides in your gut—called the gut-associated lymphoid tissue—to resolve inflammation. Protectins are derived from DHA and act as an emergency brake for the inflammatory response. In other words, when the magnitude or duration of inflammation is excessive, protectins pull the emergency brake to help normalize the inflammatory response.
- Ginger – Ginger contains potent anti-inflammatory compounds called gingerols that inhibit prostaglandin synthesis and the 5-lipoxygenase (5-LOX) enzyme.[40] The 5-LOX enzyme is responsible for the removal of arachidonic acid, but it also stimulates the

production of pro-inflammatory molecules known as leukotrienes.

- Turmeric spice – A common spice used in Indian and Thai cuisine, turmeric contains curcumin, which provides broad anti-inflammatory benefits. Like ginger, turmeric influences the 5-LOX and COX pathways that promote inflammation.[41]
- Cinnamon – Cinnamon, or one of its constituents cinnamaldehyde, helps relieve inflammation by inhibiting the release of arachidonic acid, and modifying prostaglandin and COX activity.[42,43]
- Garlic – A compound found in garlic called allicin is considered to be the active compound that produces its anti-inflammatory activity. Allicin reduces the production of pro-inflammatory cytokines and increases heme oxygenase-1 (HO-1)—an enzyme with major immunomodulatory and anti-inflammatory properties—activity.[44]
- Dark leafy greens (spinach, kale, broccoli) – These greens contain vitamin E, which alters the production of cytokines—molecules that are critical regulators of the immune and inflammatory response.[45]
- Nuts – Nuts help reduce CRP levels, inhibit interleukin-6 (IL-6)—a pro-inflammatory cytokine, and provide antioxidants to help repair damage caused by inflammation.[46]

- Olive oil – A compound found in olive oil, oleocanthal—considered by some a natural NSAID,[47] inhibits the COX pathways to reduce inflammation. In fact, about three and a half tablespoons of olive oil is equivalent to taking 200 mg of ibuprofcn (keep in mind that 3.5 tablespoons of olive oil provides about 416 calories).[48]
- Berries – Containing abundant polyphenols, like anthocyanins, berries have a strong anti-inflammatory effect in humans.[49] Anthocyanins exert their anti-inflammatory effects through moderating the COX pathways and inhibiting prostaglandins.[50]
- Tart cherries – Like berries, tart cherries are high in anthocyanins. They help decrease pain and inflammation by reducing CRP levels,[51] inhibiting the COX enzymes,[52,53] and reducing symptoms of exercise-induced muscle damage.[54]

Many AS patients experience a reduction in their symptoms by simply eliminating sugar, dairy, and gluten from their diet. These are the three most pro-inflammatory parts of the modern diet. Limit or eliminate the following foods and ingredients that may increase inflammation from your diet:
- Sugar – Sugar, in all its forms (fructose, brown sugar, cane sugar, etc.) is a highly pro-inflammatory nutrient that triggers overactivity of the immune system. Sugar

disrupts the production of proteolytic enzymes—enzymes produced by the pancreas that inhibit inflammation (even better than NSAIDs), reduce edema (by enhancing lymphatic drainage), and diminish pain.[55] Consuming excess sugar can also lead to an increased production of advanced glycation end-products (AGEs)—sugar molecules attached to proteins or lipids glycating them—triggering inflammation that has been linked to arthritis.[56]

- Dairy (cheese, milk) – Interestingly, Harvard research suggests that consuming animal products, like dairy, introduces harmful microorganisms into the gut and dramatically alters the balance of harmful to friendly bacteria that inhabit the gut.[57] Remarkably the researchers concluded that consuming animal products could alter gut microbiome balance so drastically that it could rapidly trigger inflammatory bowel disease in only two days. Casein, the chief protein found in cow's milk, is often used in studies as a pro-inflammatory agent to induce the inflammatory response.[58]

- Gluten – We are not eating the same wheat that our parents and grandparents ate. In order to improve crop yield, and make wheat more bug resistant and drought tolerant, scientists have hybridized wheat, and with it created new proteins and an imbalanced grain. One of the results is widespread gluten—a protein found in wheat, barley, and rye—intolerance and increased rates of gastrointestinal disorders. Gluten may increase the permeability of the intestines and trigger a pro-inflammatory immune response, leading to chronic inflammation, and autoinflammatory and autoimmune diseases.[59,60] This has even been suspected as a contributing factor in the development of AS.[61] One of the basic functions of intestinal cells is to regulate intestinal permeability. In predisposed or genetically susceptible individuals, gluten causes intestinal cells to release too much zonulin—a protein that regulates the permeability of tight junctions in the intestinal tract.[62] Zonulin is like a gatekeeper for the intestines, allowing or blocking nutrients and other molecules from passing through. The problem with gluten is the overstimulation and overproduction of zonulin, which causes the tight intestinal junctions to open excessively, allowing larger molecules—toxins, microbes, bacteria, gluten peptides, and other harmful substances—to enter the bloodstream. This leakage of larger molecules creates an immune cascade that encourages autoinflammatory and autoimmune disorders.[63] Gluten also accelerates the production of inflammatory cytokines.[64] Eliminating gluten from the diet is associated with improved insulin response, reduced obesity, and decreased inflammation.[65] Substitute gluten free grains like amaranth, buckwheat, corn, millet, quinoa, rice, sorghum, and non-contaminated oats instead.

- Saturated and trans fats – Consuming saturated fat is linked to the increased expression of pro-inflammatory genes in adipose tissue—body tissue used for the storage of fat.[66] Trans fats similarly stimulate a pro-inflammatory response.[67]
- Omega-6 essential fatty acids (EFAs) – Some omega-6 EFAs promote inflammation, and if not enough omega-3 EFAs are present to balance them, the inflammatory process in the body may increase. One study found that the optimal ratio of omega-6 to omega-3 EFAs to suppress inflammation in patients with rheumatoid arthritis is 2 or 3 to 1.[68]
- Refined carbohydrates – Eating excess refined carbohydrates can produce an acute inflammatory response in adipose tissue that eventually becomes chronic.[69] Reducing refined carbohydrates is of particular importance if you experience inflammatory bowel diseases like Crohn's disease.[70] Excess consumption of refined carbohydrates is associated with an almost three-fold increase in inflammatory disease mortality.[71] Dr. Alan Ebringer, professor of immunology at King's College London, believes that starches should

be particularly avoided with AS because they can trigger a complex immune response involving the growth and perpetuation of pathogenic organisms in the gut, thus triggering or exacerbating disease process. Research does exist that supports this theory, with findings suggesting that starch-containing products lead to an increased presence of the pathogen *Klebsiella pneumonia*, which subsequently increases production of antibodies to this pathogen, as well as autoantibodies that damage the bowel and joints.[72,73] Eating less starch-containing foods—potatoes, grains, and baked goods—and replacing them with non-starchy carbohydrates—vegetables and fruits—could result in a reduction of inflammation and AS symptoms.[74]

- Meat – Besides introducing harmful bacteria into the gut and destabilizing the gut microbiome balance, meat consumption is associated with an increase in inflammatory markers and unfavorable glucose control responses.[75] This is quite a dilemma because poor glucose control accelerates the inflammatory response and negatively affects the immune system.[76] Much of the increase in inflammatory markers was attributed to an increase in body mass index (BMI). It is important to note that any foods that promote weight gain or obesity should be eaten cautiously because extra weight places an increased burden on the joints. Interestingly, German physicians reported that an HLA-B27 positive patient with sacroiliitis—inflammation of the sacroiliac joint common to AS—experienced significant improvement of symptoms (pain and morning stiffness) three to four days after switching to a vegan diet.[77] When the patient reverted to eating meat six weeks later symptoms worsened, so the patient switched back to a vegan diet. After three months of follow-up the physicians observed that the patient was almost completely free of symptoms, no longer required tramadol and ibuprofen, and had halved the dosage of meloxicam required for pain relief.

If you experience a flare-up in symptoms, it may be beneficial to temporarily eliminate gluten, dairy, meat, and processed sugar from your diet for a few days or until symptoms are relieved. This will eliminate potential triggers of the flare-up and allow your body to reset and heal.

One of the simplest, yet effective ways to reduce joint pain is to drink adequate amounts of water every day. Maintaining sufficient water intake may reduce pain and stiffness, increase nutrient transport to the joints, and help lubricate the joints. Strive to drink half of your body weight in ounces each day (i.e. if you are 120 pounds you would drink 60 ounces of clean filtered water daily).

Remember, nutrition is the foundation of your health and eating better can improve the effectiveness of virtually all of the other strategies that you will undertake to manage AS. It is better to make small changes in your eating behaviors rather than drastic alterations. As you adjust to a different approach to eating you may experience some stomach discomfort, headaches, or general malaise. Don't worry, as this is normal and if you push through it you are likely to feel better on the other side.

Physical Activity and Ankylosing Spondylitis

Staying physically active despite some discomfort is vital to managing AS, and one of the single most important things you can do to help yourself. Careful regular physical activity, stretching, and flexibility exercises will increase your fitness and flexibility, leading to a reduction in painful, stiff, and swollen joints. You may need to experiment with what time of day is best for you to exercise. For some, midday or in the evening may be the only time the pain and stiffness is diminished enough to exercise. Others may find that moving in the morning despite the pain helps. Always consult with your physician to ensure you are healthy enough to participate in physical activity before beginning any exercise program.

Some of the benefits of regular physical activity for AS patients include:
- Improved pain tolerance.
- Reduced stiffness.
- Better flexibility and improved range of motion to make everyday tasks easier. If your back is very stiff and painful, even putting your socks or pants on can be challenging.
- Enhanced sleep quality.
- Improved lung capacity.
- Better posture.

- Enhanced balance.
- Improved cardiovascular fitness.
- Stronger muscles and bones.
- A more balanced mood.
- Better immune system function.

Many AS patients find that swimming is an enjoyable, low-impact activity to improve general fitness, flexibility, and strength. According to the U.K. National Ankylosing Spondylitis Society, the best stroke for AS patients is the front crawl, followed by the back crawl.[78] They recommend avoiding the butterfly and breast strokes because they put excess strain on the back and neck, and may inflame the hips and pelvis. Light water aerobics is also a good option.

When you have sore joints or a sore back, strength training may seem too painful to participate in, but it is critical to maintain bone and muscle health. You need strong muscles to support your joints properly, and strong bones to reduce the risk of osteopenia and osteoporosis. Those with ankylosing spondylitis are more prone to bone mineral loss, particularly of the femoral head and spine, which may lead to osteoporosis.[79,80] Strength training increases bone mineral density, therefore improving bone health and reducing the risk of fractures. It is especially important to strengthen the abdominals, back, and muscles between the shoulder blades.

Unless you have fused vertebrae or a rod inserted in your spine, it is not usually necessary to limit the weight that you use during strength training. In fact, I participate in high-intensity metabolic resistance training three times per week. Others find that they are able to lift the same weight they used to before they were diagnosed with AS. Talk to your doctor about your current state of health and what you are able to participate in, but keep moving.

A number of studies suggest that yoga is very beneficial for reducing back pain, decreasing functional limitations, and even diminishing the need for pain medication.[81,82,83,84] Indeed, yoga may be more beneficial than other forms of exercise when it comes to relieving pain.[85] Scientists have discovered that participating in yoga increases brain-derived neurotrophic factor (BDNF)[86]—a secreted protein that is influential in the nervous system's response to pain and a person's pain tolerance level—and helps maintain serotonin levels, which will benefit mood.

One particular form of yoga to consider is Iyengar yoga, which emphasizes precision and alignment in all postures. This particular yoga practice is associated with significant reductions in pain intensity, functional disability, and pain medication use among patients with chronic low back pain.[87]

The great thing about yoga is that virtually anyone can participate in it at some level because there are beginner, intermediate, and advanced levels, as well as modified versions of the postures. I practice yoga twice per week and find it very useful in relieving my AS symptoms.

Stretching and flexibility exercises are vital to managing AS because they improve range of motion and reduce joint stiffness and pain. They are so vital that I do them—and suggest others do as well—every day. Your stretching and flexibility plan should include exercises that strengthen your core. I find that doing some gentle back stretches just prior to going to bed makes a big difference in the amount of pain and stiffness I feel when I wake up. I also perform regular back and core exercises during the day.

I have found the following exercises to strengthen and support my back and relieve pain and stiffness. You should have your current level of pain, flexibility, disease progression, and overall health evaluated by a physician before beginning any of these exercises.

Just prior to going to bed I perform one or both of the following—Cat & Cow and Alternating Up Dog and Down Dog.

CAT & COW
Benefits:
- Stretches the back, hips, chest and abdominals.
- Strengthens the lower back, hip muscles, and abdominals.
- Increases the flexibility and function of the spine.

- Decrease pain and stiffness in the lower back.

How to Perform: Get down on your hands and knees with your palms flat on the floor about shoulder distance apart and your knees about hip distance apart. Keep your back flat and head relaxed. Round your back up toward the ceiling (Cat) until you feel a stretch in your entire back. Hold the stretch for about 10 seconds. Return to the starting position and then press your stomach toward the floor while lifting your buttocks towards the ceiling (Cow). Hold this position for ten seconds. Repeat the process three to five times.

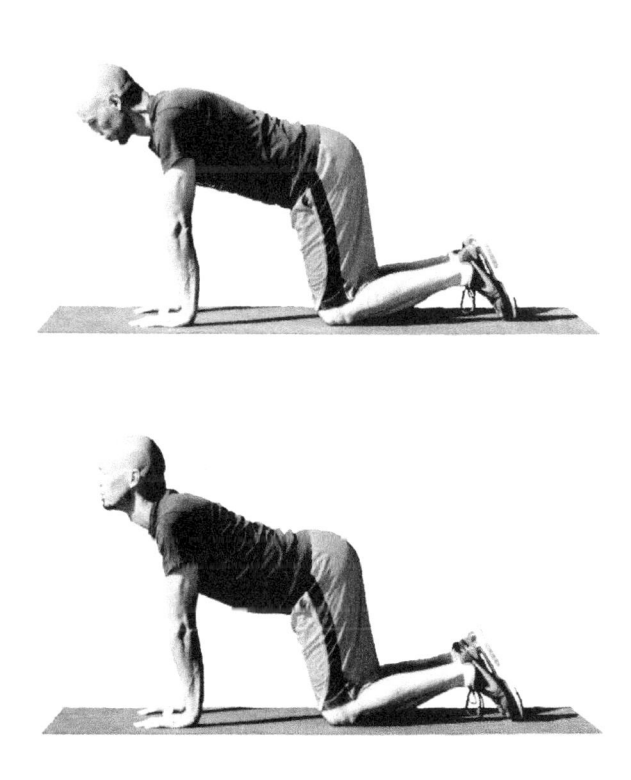

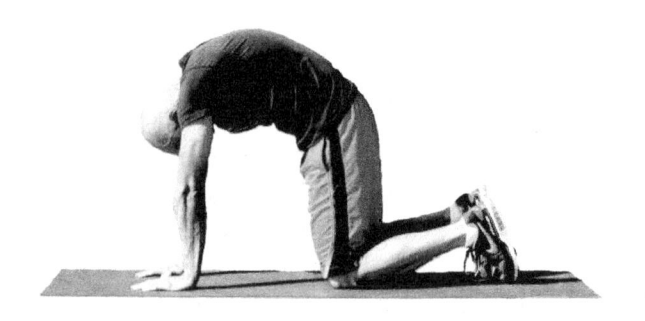

UP DOG & DOWN DOG (MODIFIED UP DOG)

May be difficult for some and cause increased back pain. Transition from Up Dog to Down Dog smoothly and in a controlled manner to avoid compression of the lumbar spine.

Benefits:
- Stretches and strengthens the chest, shoulders, back, and abdomen.
- Increases the flexibility of the spine.
- Firms buttocks.

How to Perform: Lie on your stomach with your toes pointed behind you, forehead flat on the ground, and legs close together. Place your palms on the floor under your shoulders (fingers spread apart). Push up with your hands keeping your elbows tight to your torso as you take a deep breath. Lean your head back and raise your torso until your arms are extended (Up Dog). Hold torso off the ground for about five to seven seconds. Exhale as you slowly lower your chest back towards the ground and lift your buttocks and hips towards the ceiling so you form an upside down V (Down Dog). Press back strongly with your arms, relax your neck, and let your head drop. You may need to bend your knees so the stretch is more in your back then your hamstrings. Hold for five to seven seconds. Rest before repeating. Perform about 10 repetitions.

Modified Up Dog: Lie on your stomach with your toes pointed behind you, forehead flat on the ground, and legs close together. Place your forearms and hands on the floor with your elbows under your shoulders (fingers spread apart, palms down). Push up leaving your forearms and hands flat on the ground raising your torso as you take a deep breath. Lean your head back and keep your torso raised for a count of about five to seven seconds then move into Down Dog.

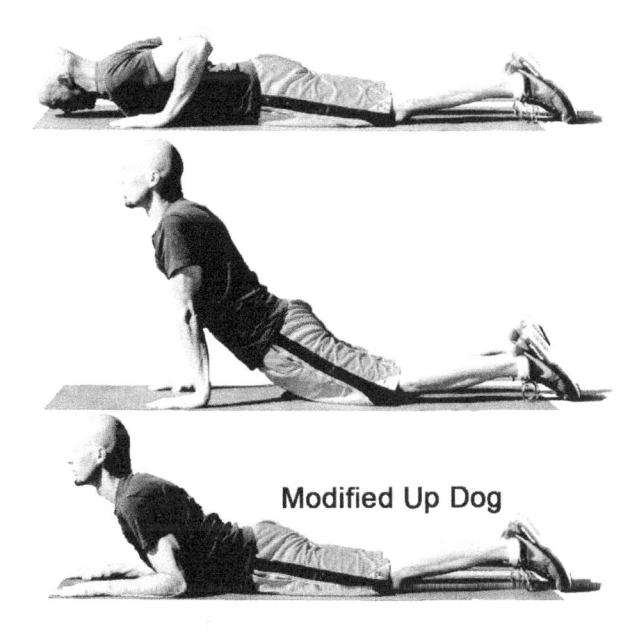

Modified Up Dog

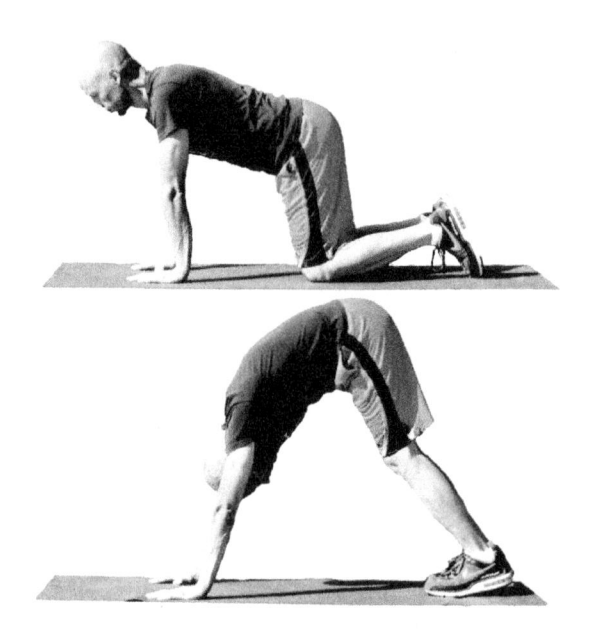

Perform this series of exercises at least three to four times weekly, preferably daily.

Pointer Dog
Benefits: <ul><li>Helps stabilize the lumbar spine.</li><li>Builds endurance and control in the back extensors.</li><li>Strengthens the glutes, abdominals, lower back, and hips.</li></ul>
How to Perform: Start on your hands and knees keeping a neutral spine. Hands should be underneath your shoulders and knees under your hips. Engage your abdominals as you simultaneously raise your left arm and right leg to extended and straight positions. Hold this position for three to five seconds. Return to the starting position. Engage your abdominals again and this time raise your right arm and your left leg to the

extended and straight positions. Hold this position for three to five seconds. Return to the starting position. Repeat the exercise 10 times on each side.

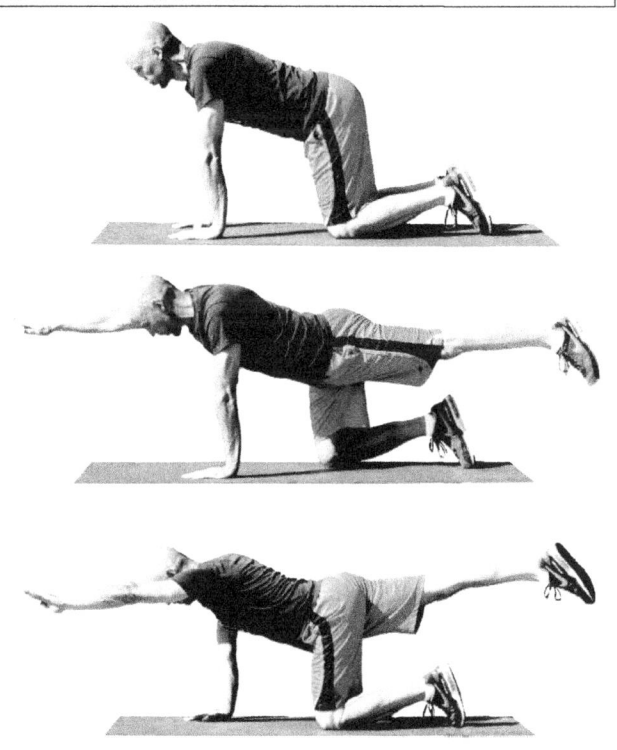

Floor Bridge
Benefits:
- Strengthens and tones the glutes, abdominals, and quadriceps and to a lesser extent erector spinae muscles—a muscle that helps straighten the back and allows side-to-side rotation.
- Builds pelvic floor strength.
- Engages inactive glutes.
- Helps stabilize your spine and reduce the

risk of back pain and hip injury.

How to Perform: Lie on your back with your knees bent at about a 45-degree angle and your feet flat on the ground about one foot in front of your buttocks. Your palms should be facing down on the floor next to your buttocks. Engage your abdominals and glutes and slowly thrust your hips upwards toward the ceiling until you create a straight line from your shoulders to your knees. Hold the bridge for two seconds then lower to the starting position. Repeat the exercise 20 to 30 times. Alternately, hold the bridge for five seconds each time and repeat 10 to 12 times.

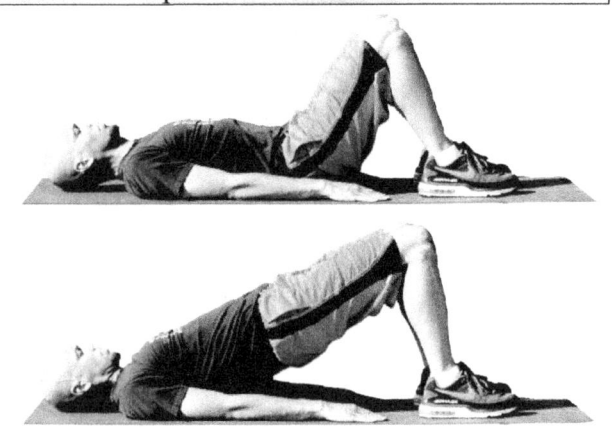

Dead Bug

Benefits:
- Strengthens the abdominals.
- Improves hand-leg coordination.
- Helps relieve low back pain.

How to Perform: Lie flat on your back with your knees bent at a 90 degree angle and calves parallel to the floor. Suck your belly button in towards your spine and simultaneously extend your left leg and your right arm (over your head). Return to the start position. Suck your belly button in towards your spine again and simultaneously extend your right leg and your left arm. Repeat the exercise on both sides 8 to 10 times and perform two to three sets.

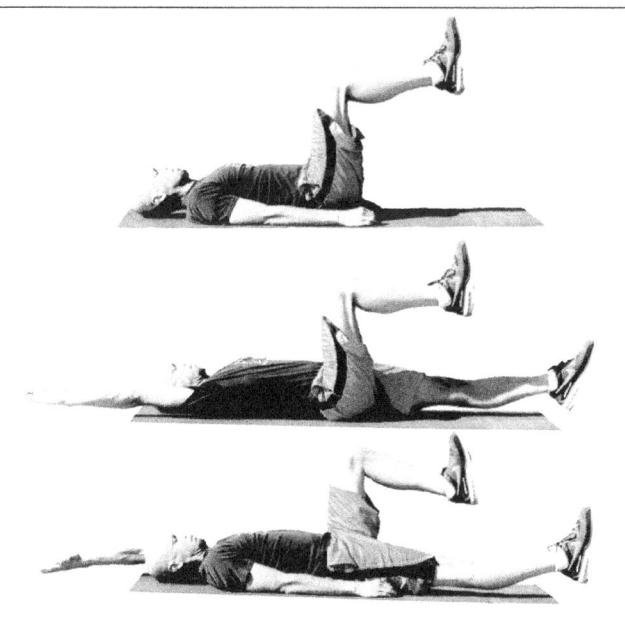

Reverse Curl Up
Benefits:
- Strengthens the abdominals without hurting your neck and back.
- Improves pelvic floor strength.
- Aids proper breathing.

How to Perform: Lie on your back with your knees and hips bent at a 90 degree angle so your calves are parallel to the floor. Your palms should be face down and extended. As you exhale, pull your knees towards your chin until your buttocks is slightly raised off the floor and your knees are close to your chest. Hold for about one to two seconds. Inhale as you return to the start position. Repeat 10 times and complete three sets.

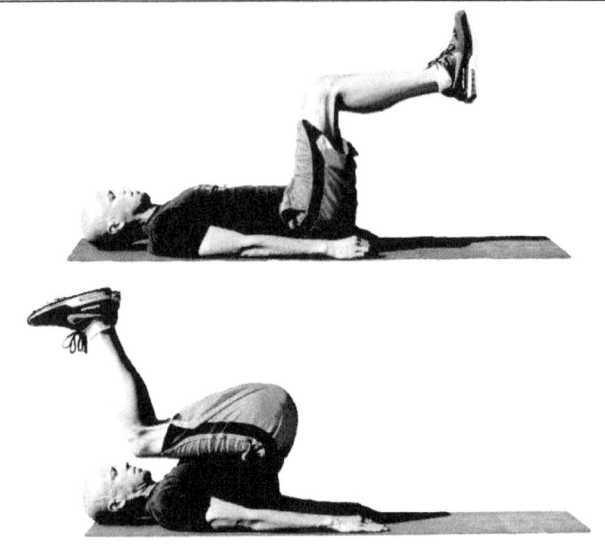

Seated Reverse Crunch

Benefits:
- Strengthens your abdominals and obliques without engaging the back or neck.
- Tones legs.
- Improves coordination and balance.
- May correct posture problems.

How to Perform: Sit at the edge of a stable chair and grip both sides of the underside of the chair with your hands for support. Slowly lean back until your back is at a 45 degree angle and straighten your legs out in front of you. Draw your knees into your chest and then return to the start position. Repeat this action for about 30 seconds and perform three sets.

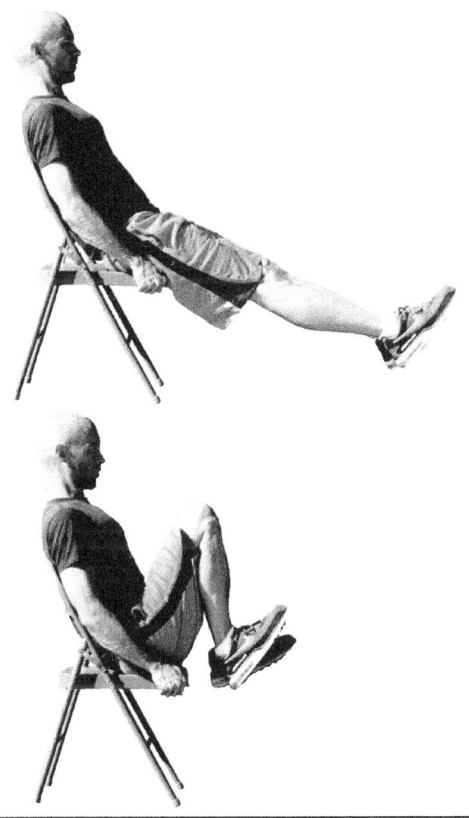

Physio Ball Single Leg Bridge

Benefits:
- Strengthens and tones the glutes, abdominals, and hamstrings.
- Increases stability and balance.
- Helps stabilize your spine and reduce the risk of back pain and injury.

How to Perform: Start in the glute bridge position with your shoulders on the physio ball and feet flat on the floor forming a straight line from your shoulders to your knees. Place your hands on your hips and slowly raise one leg to the straight and extended position without letting the other hip drop down. Hold this position for 5 to 10 seconds then slowly lower your leg. Repeat the process with the other leg and complete 5 to 10 repetitions with each leg.

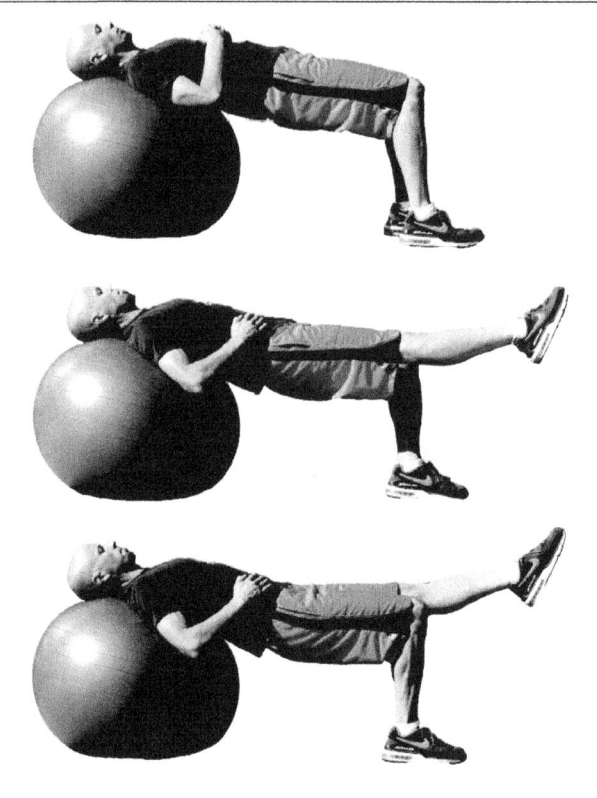

These exercises are more advanced core and back exercises that should not be performed until you are comfortable with the above exercises.

Superman/Superwoman Over a Physio Ball
Benefits:
• Develops your core.
• Strengthens the lower and middle back, shoulders, hamstrings, and glutes.
• Encourages good balance.

How to Perform: Get down on your knees with your feet flat against a sturdy wall and the physio ball positioned directly in front of you and against your pelvis. Lean down on the ball and tighten your legs as you roll straight forward so your body is in a straight position and your hands are down next to your side. Keep your head straight (in line with your spine) and face down. As you progress you can reach your hands out forward. Hold the position for 20 to 30 seconds and repeat three to four times.

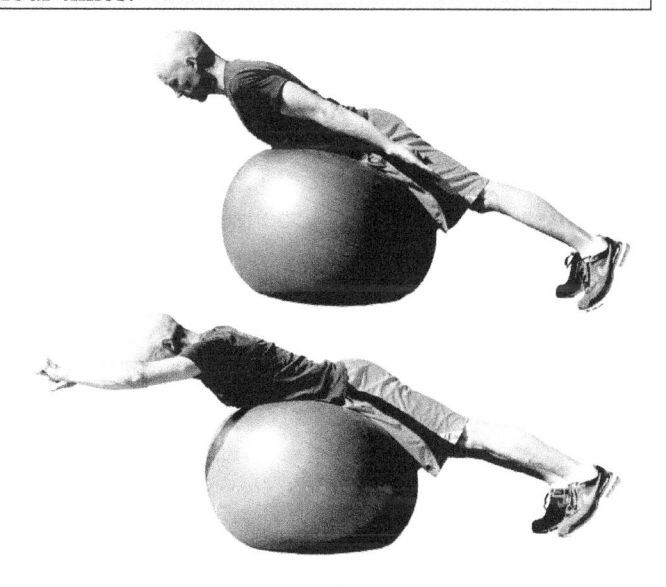

Plank (Forearm or Standard)

This exercise could potentially exacerbate low back pain and should only be performed by those who have strengthened their core and back with the other exercises first.

Benefits:
- Strengthens and tones the shoulders, biceps, chest, abdominals, glutes, legs, and back.
- Improves shoulder girdle, back, and leg

flexibility.
- Elongates the body and counteracts a weak back.

How to Perform: Start in the pushup position (hands directly beneath your shoulders forming a straight line from your heels to the tip of your head). Hold this position for 30 to 60 seconds and then slowly lower to the ground. Repeat three times.

Forearm Plank: Start in the pushup position. Bend your elbows 90 degrees so that your forearms are flat on the ground and your elbows are directly beneath your shoulders. Make sure your body forms a straight line from your heels to the tip of your head). Hold this position for 30 to 60 seconds then slowly lower to the ground. Repeat three times.

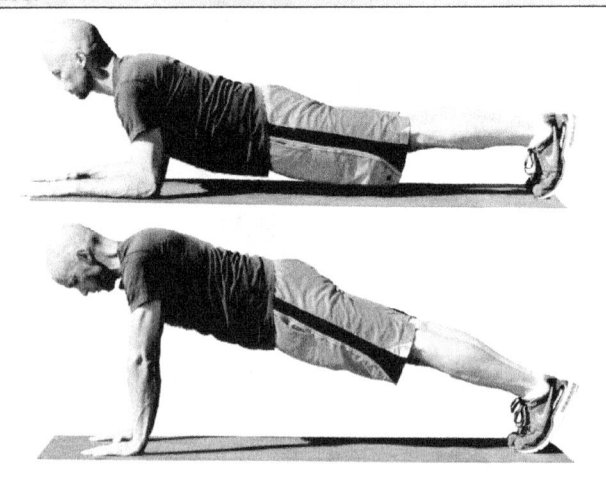

Side Plank Over a Physio Ball (Hip on ball)
Challenging. May need to work up to this.

Benefits:
- Strengthens your core, particularly your

> obliques and quadratus lumborum.
> - Reduces the risk of low back pain.

How to Perform: Place your feet against the wall staggered one in front of the other. Place the physio ball underneath your hip and raise your body up so that you create a straight line from your feet against the wall to your head. Place your hand closest to the ball on the ground and your other hand on you hip. For a more advanced version, fold your arms across your chest while holding the exercise. Hold for 15 to 30 seconds, working up to 30 or 60 seconds. Repeat the exercise twice on each side.

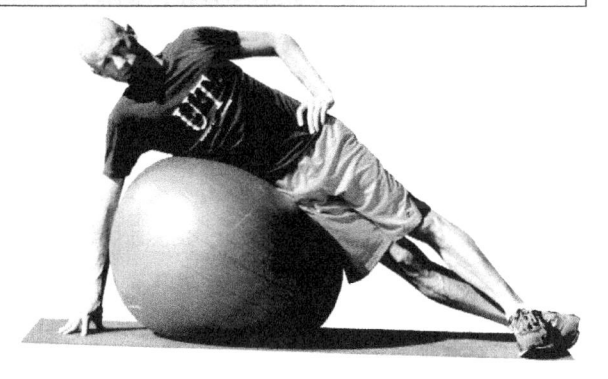

To support muscle health and avoid muscle atrophy and/or wasting, it is essential to supply the body with adequate protein. Much of your protein requirements can be obtained through diet. If not, whey or vegetarian protein supplements are also available. Aim for 1 to 1.5 g/kg of body weight.

AS and Intimacy

Research has discovered that the chronic nature, pain, and functional ability of AS may make sexual activity more challenging.[88,89,90] However, research also suggests that sexual enjoyment and frequency of orgasms are similar to those without AS when sexual activity is possible.

It is important to find ways to enjoy intimacy with your spouse, and adjustments may be necessary on both partners' part. Share your limitations with your spouse and what you would like to do to stay sexually active. Positions can be adapted so that you feel less pain, are better supported, and remain comfortable. Intimacy releases hormones that elevate your pain threshold and may even provide temporary relief from the pain. Not to mention, intimacy is a great mood booster.

Most physicians will tell you to avoid high-impact activities—running, basketball, football, rugby, hockey, wrestling—due to an increased risk of injury. It is true that these activities do cause extra stress on the joints and spine and may increase your risk of injury, but I have found that I am able to enjoy many of the activities I did before my diagnosis—basketball, football (flag or two-hand touch), and some running. Collaborate with your physician and determine which activities are best for you and avoid those that you know aggravate symptoms. For example, I have found that running during sports is tolerable, but running steadily for greater distances aggravates my symptoms so I avoid it.

Natural Remedies for Ankylosing Spondylitis

Since AS is a multifaceted and highly adaptable disease it requires a multidimensional approach with natural remedies. Your management plan may include remedies that protect the joints, heart, eyes, and lungs, reduce inflammation and pain, and support the immune and gastrointestinal systems. The results you experience will depend largely on disease progression, medications that you take, your current state of health, and how early after diagnosis supplementary measures are started—the earlier the better.

Foundational Nutrients
The foundation of an AS dietary supplement plan should include an optimum potency multi-nutrient (a multivitamin, multi-mineral supplement with other beneficial phytonutrients). People with chronic illnesses require more nutrients than those without them, and so providing your body essential vitamins, minerals, and other nutrients is key. Evidence suggests that AS patients have lower levels of several key antioxidants including beta carotene, vitamins A, C, and E, and reduced glutathione (GSH).[91] Choose a multi-nutrient that provides at least the recommended daily allowance of most of the nutrients listed on the label, but more is even better. Taking an optimum

potency multi-nutrient daily will help provide any nutrients that may be deficient and contributing to disease progression and intensity.

Another important foundational nutrient is a high-quality, molecularly distilled marine oil supplement. Research suggests that omega-3 essential fatty acids, like those found in marine sources, may influence AS disease activity.[92,93] Omega-3s help normalize inflammation, and reduce inflammatory cytokines, T-lymphocyte activation—excess production is a contributing factor to immune-associated arthritis—and catabolic enzymes—enzymes involved in the perception of pain.

Marine omega-3 fatty acids, DHA and EPA, are essential for the production of two compounds that control inflammation—resolvins and protectins—and inhibit TNF-β.[94] These anti-inflammatory compounds help maintain a normal inflammatory response and put a brake on inflammation when it becomes excessive. In addition, omega-3s help protect your cardiovascular system.[95]

A clinical trial investigating the effects of supplementing omega-3 fatty acids in AS patients reported some promising findings. Study participants in the trial that received 4.55 grams of omega-3 fatty acids daily experienced a significant reduction in disease activity.[96] Strive for 2 to 5 grams of marine fish oil daily, supplying a total of at least 500 mg each of DHA and EPA.

Emerging research suggests that a substantial amount of AS disease progression—and autoinflammatory conditions for that matter—centers around the gut. This makes taking a high-potency, clinically-proven multi-strain probiotic absolutely essential. It is well-known that probiotics support healthy digestion and elimination, but few realize the far-reaching benefits for the whole body that they provide. Research suggests that probiotics provide protection from infectious diseases, help normalize inflammation, support the immune system and influence mood and behavior. They also provide protection from autoimmune and inflammatory diseases and support a healthy mucosal barrier in the gut.[97]

Scientists have discovered that probiotics—specifically the *L. casei* 01 strain—decrease inflammatory cytokines, overall inflammation, and improve disease activity in patients with rheumatoid arthritis.[98] *Lactobacillus reuteri* RC-14, *Lactobacillus rhamnosus* GR-1,[99] *Lactobacillus rhamnosus* GG,[100] and *Lactobacillus casei* (by inhibiting COX-2)[101] have also demonstrated anti-inflammatory activity in patients with arthritis. Lastly, probiotics help alleviate the inflammatory bowel diseases associated with AS.[102] Aim for at least 8 billion viable organisms daily, with a probiotic feeder like free oligosaccharides (FOS), preferably including one or more of the strains listed above.

Targeted Nutrients

A potent antioxidant that significantly reduces pain and inflammation, turmeric, is a powerful tool for AS patients. It thwarts inflammation by inhibiting COX-2, prostaglandins, leukotrienes, and cytokines involved in the initiation and progression of inflammation.[103,104,105,106] In addition, one of the primary compounds in turmeric, curcumin, has demonstrated the ability to protect against various pro-inflammatory diseases by down-regulating TNF-α.[107,108] Turmeric is often standardized for curcuminoids, or the curcumin is used alone.

An animal study found that administration of turmeric prevented the degeneration of bone and joints in collagen-induced arthritis (CIA) rats.[109] CIA models are often used in animals to simulate the immunological and pathological effects of human rheumatoid arthritis. A human trial comparing a lecithin form of curcumin with acetaminophen and nimesulide—a relatively selective COX-2 inhibiting NSAID—concluded that 2 grams of curcumin provided the equivalent pain and inflammation relief as compared to 1 gram of acetaminophen, but did not work as well as nimesulide.[110]

Curcumin is not readily absorbed, but absorption can be improved by taking it with food.[111] The therapeutic dosage should be between 500 and 1,000 mg twice daily. Turmeric should not be taken with anticoagulant or antiplatelet drugs due to potential interactions.

Used as a medicinal herb for centuries, ginger is a powerful anti-inflammatory and pain reliever. It is a natural COX-2[112] and 5-LOX[113] inhibitor, and decreases leukotrienes,[114] TNF-α,[115] and prostaglandins[116] involved in inflammation and the perception of pain. With its multiple mechanisms of action, ginger should be part of your daily regimen to control pain and inflammation.

Unlike drugs that only attack AS symptoms such as inflammation and pain, ginger actually helps to reduce bone destruction.[117] Ginger essential oil can also be applied topically to relieve pain. A study combining massage with topical application of ginger essential oil reported that subjects with chronic lower back pain experienced short- and long-term pain and disability relief from the practice.[118] Depending on the extract used, therapeutic doses of ginger range from 170 to 255 mg three times daily. Ginger could potentially interact with blood-thinners, antidiabetes, and cholesterol medications.

A naturally occurring compound and metabolite of dimethylsulfoxide (DMSO), the organic sulfur compound methylsulfonylmethane (MSM), may inhibit degenerative changes to joints and helps stabilize cell membranes—keeps them permeable so nutrients can enter the cell and waste can exit, and scavenge proinflammatory free-radicals.[119,120] MSM is often combined with glucosamine and chondroitin, as it improves the efficacy of each individual nutrient.[121] Glucosamine and chondroitin are both building blocks for a molecule called glycosaminoglycan—a molecule used by the body to produce and repair cartilage. Research suggests that glucosamine and chondroitin protect cartilage and help repair degeneration of spinal discs.[122,123] These nutrients may support healthy joints and joint cartilage, as well as reduce the risk of osteoporosis and fractures associated with AS.

Some research suggests that these three nutrients—particularly glucosamine—are less effective or ineffective when taken alone, so they should always be taken together. MSM is considered a very safe nutrient and even extreme dosages—8 grams per kg of body weight per day—have not produced toxicity.[124] Therapeutic dosages range from 500 mg three times daily to 3,000 mg twice daily. Glucosamine is usually taken at 500 mg three times daily in combination with 400 mg of chondroitin three times daily. Both glucosamine and chondroitin may increase the blood thinning effects of anticoagulant medications.

While the name may conjure memories of eating black licorice candy, deglycyrrhizinated licorice (DGL) is much more than a sweet treat. DGL has most of the glycyrrhizin and glycyrrhetinic acids removed to eliminate the blood pressure raising effect seen in the whole herb. This is one of my favorite medicinal herbs because it is so effective with stomach problems, and I personally used it to heal an indomethacin-induced ulcer.

DGL offers broad benefits to AS sufferers, serving four distinct purposes. First, it helps maintain the protective mucosal lining of the stomach—and repairs it when it is damaged—helping to reduce a very common side effect of NSAIDs.[125] This occurs without the suppression of gastric acid production, which is what many drugs with a similar purpose do. Therefore, those who suffer with heartburn, peptic ulcers, or indigestion can find great relief with DGL. Although research has focused on DGL's effect on the upper gastrointestinal system, DGL also travels to the lower intestinal tract and may influence intestinal permeability. DGL is a demulcent—a substance that relieves mucosal inflammation and irritation by forming a protective barrier, and therefore could potentially heal the entire gastrointestinal system.

Secondly, DGL helps to reduce the duration and severity of canker sores.[126] I found this by chance as I was taking DGL daily to repair my ulcer. I noticed that I was no longer experiencing any canker sores. After my ulcer healed, I quit taking DGL and I experienced a canker sore cropping up here and there. I have placed a DGL tablet directly on a canker sore to aid the healing process and find it effective in reducing pain, duration, and severity of canker sores.

Third, DGL is believed to create a favorable environment—by supporting gastrointestinal health and discouraging harmful bacteria—for healthy bacteria to flourish within the gut. Improved gut microbiome may enhance the immune system, help normalize the inflammatory response, and reduce inflammatory bowel diseases.

Lastly, DGL supports the endocrine system, particularly influencing adrenal gland function to reduce fatigue. It slows down the breakdown of essential hormones and improves the body's response to cortisol,[127] which may help relieve pain, weakness, cognitive impairment, and chronic fatigue often associated with adrenal fatigue or dysfunction.

The usual dose of DGL is 380 to 400 mg in the form of a chewable tablet taken 20 minutes before each meal. Although the glycyrrhizin and glycyrrhetinic acids have been removed, if you experience any swelling of the ankles or increase in blood pressure, you should discontinue DGL usage to determine if this improves symptoms. If it does then DGL is likely a causal factor.

Boswellia serrata extracts (BSE) or boswellic acids (BA), obtained from the gum resin of frankincense trees, possess anti-inflammatory, anti-arthritis, and pain-relieving properties. Some boswellic acids (acetyl-11-keto-boswellic acids, AKBA) inhibit 5-LOX, while others inhibit TNF-α or leukotrienes, without side effects.[128,129,130] With these properties BSE and BAs have demonstrated positive effects on common chronic inflammatory diseases like rheumatoid arthritis, bronchial asthma, osteoarthritis, ulcerative colitis, and Crohn's disease.[131] In addition, BAs may modify immune responses associated with autoinflammatory and autoimmune disorders.[132,133] Typical dosages range from 300 mg three times daily to 3,600 mg per day. It is possible for BAs to interact with immunosuppressant medications and drugs metabolized by the cytochrome P450 pathway.

Enzymes are proteins that facilitate chemical reactions necessary for the proper function of tissues, muscles, bones, organs, and cells. Proteolytic enzymes, or proteases, breakdown peptide bonds in protein foods to release amino acids. Examples include pepsin, bromelain (from pineapples), papain (from papayas), trypsin, and chrymotrypsin. In addition to their function in proteolysis, proteolytic enzymes have been investigated for their benefits for a number of conditions such as cancer, autoimmune disorders, and chronic inflammatory conditions.

Proteolytic enzymes help combat inflammation by regulating the inflammatory response, moderating protease-activated receptors—receptors that trigger a response to injury, including inflammation, pain, and repair mechanisms—and by controlling the release of cytokines.[134,135] By mediating both pain and inflammation, proteolytic enzymes may help manage the symptoms of AS.

Essential oils are potent natural remedies that can be administered topically, orally, and inhaled to help manage AS. A number of essential oils possess powerful anti-inflammatory or analgesic (pain relieving) properties.

Taking into account the possible connection between dormant pathogenic organisms—*Klebsiella pneumoniae, Staphylococci, and E. coli*—the topical application of essential oils to the spine may also combat disease progression related to microbes.

Cypress (*Cupressus sempervirens*) actively inhibits *K. pneumoniae*,[136] relieves muscle spasms, and aids the circulatory system. Tea tree oil (*Melaleuca alternifolia*) is effective against gram-negative bacteria like *E. coli* and *K. pneumonia*,[137] and is a mild anti-inflammatory. Peppermint (*Mentha piperita*), basil (*Ocimum basilicum*), oregano (*Origanum vulgare*), and marjoram (*Origanum majorana*) are all strong inhibitors of *K. pneumoniae*,[138] some inhibit *E. coli*,[139,140,141] and they all help relieve pain and/or inflammation. Geranium (*Pelargonium graveolens*) is anti-inflammatory, supports the nervous and endocrine systems, and inhibits both *K. pneumoniae* and *Staphylococci*.[142,143] The eucalyptus essential oils are antimicrobial, anti-inflammatory, support the respiratory system, and relieve joint and muscle pain. *Eucalyptus globulus* inhibits both *E. coli* and *Staphylococci*.[144] Cinnamon, thyme, and clove also inhibit *K. pneumoniae*.[145] Lemongrass and oregano inhibit both *K. pneumoniae* and *E. coli*.[146]

By applying a combination of these essential oils to the spine, you could affect a number of AS symptoms, including pain, inflammation, and dysfunction, combat potentially pathogenic organisms, and support the gastrointestinal system. It is best to apply the oils diluted in a carrier oil—preferably aloe vera for its anti-inflammatory and digestive supporting properties. St. John's Wort carrier oil can also be used because it provides additional anti-inflammatory properties for sciatica and nerve damage, but it is contraindicated during pregnancy, or when taking antidepressants, anticoagulants, antiplatelet medications, tramadol, drug contraceptives, and protease inhibitors. A good ratio for dilution is 5 to 30 drops of essential oil to 5 ml of carrier oil—start at the lower end until your body is accustomed to the essential oils. Do not apply the essential oils daily for more than three consecutive weeks without taking a one-week break. Some essential oils may interact with pain medications and/or other medications, and so it is best to reduce the number of drops by half and apply or take essential oils at least four hours after medications.

If you want to take essential oils internally you could consider taking 3 drops each of copaiba, ginger, frankincense, and balsam fir a few times daily. To encourage optimum red blood cell production, take a capsule with 5 to 10 drops of lemon oil daily also. Lastly, citrus essential oils that contain significant quantities of limonene are known to help the body produce its own antioxidants—particularly glutathione.[147] Glutathione (GSH) is often deficient in AS patients as are several other key antioxidants.

Homeopathic Remedies

Rhus toxicodendron (*Rhus tox* for short) is a homeopathic remedy derived from the poison ivy plant. Don't worry, it is diluted so heavily that virtually none of the poison ivy plant remains, leaving only the healing essence of the plant in the remedy. It is a remedy often used for rheumatism, pain, and stiffness after rest that improves from limbering and warmth. It benefits several body systems including the joints, eyes, and mucous membranes. While generally not curative in nature, it can help manage AS symptoms and reduce pain and stiffness. It is commonly taken as a sublingual tablet, though topical creams and gels also exist.

Other homeopathic remedies that may be useful, and are often blended together to make a combination remedy for mild to moderate arthritis, pain, and inflammation include *Kali Carbonicum, Natrum muriaticum, Sulphur, Silicea, Sepia,* and *Pulsatilla. Kali Carbonicum* is usually deep acting and particularly useful for lower back pain that extends down into the buttocks and back of the legs. One combination remedy I have found effective is Zeel®, Heel BHI, Arthritis Pain Relief, which is indicated for mild joint pain and stiffness.

A prized homeopathic remedy for sore muscles, sprains, and bruises, *Arnica montana* is worth mentioning for relief from inflamed tendons and muscle aches associated with AS. Some animal and clinical studies suggest arnica may control both pain and inflammation similarly to NSAIDS for some specific conditions.[148] It too, comes in sublingual tablet or topical form. Both the oral and topical forms work amazingly for muscle soreness and inflamed tendons.

Topical Analgesics
Some natural topical pain relievers have already been mentioned, but there are a few more worth considering that may provide relief of AS symptoms. They include capsaicin, and some brand name products that I have found useful—Topricin®, Cristopher's Original Formulas® Complete Tissue & Bone Ointment, and Triflora®. I generally use these for flare-ups rather than daily usage.

An active component of chili peppers, capsaicin works by warming and irritating the tissues to release substance P[149]—a chemical that is ordinarily released when tissues are damaged. With repeated applications substance P becomes depleted in that location, relieving pain in the area of application. Capsaicin also modifies nociceptor—nerve cell endings that initiate the sensation of pain by sending signals to the spinal cord and brain—activity.[150] It has been found to be very effective for chronic musculoskeletal pain.[151]

Topricin® is indicated for a number of symptoms associated with AS, like arthritis, joint diseases, back pain, tendonitis, and sciatica. Triflora® is suggested for back pain, rheumatism, arthritis, and tendinitis.

Cristopher's Original Formulas® Complete Tissue & Bone Ointment contains a combination of herbs that helps relieve bruises, stiff necks, sprains, and symptoms of arthritis, and encourages the healing of bones and cartilage. They are all worth trying and usually need to be applied three to several times daily to maintain relief.

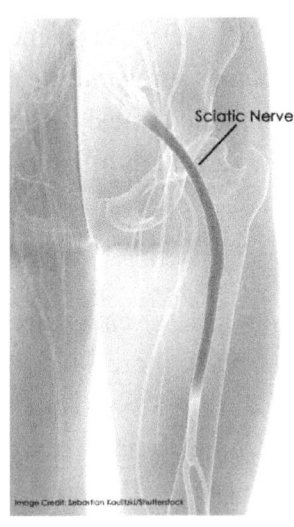

Other Remedies

AS is a very adaptive and progressive disease, so a variety of remedies will likely need to be employed and rotated to avoid building up a tolerance and allowing AS to adapt to them thus decreasing their effectiveness. Other natural anti-inflammatory substances include guggul, vitamin D and astaxanthin. Another nutrient that is beneficial for AS is vitamin C.

Guggul, derived from Indian frankincense (*Boswellia serrata*) oleo-gum resin has been used in Ayurvedic medicine for thousands of years and possesses anti-inflammatory activity,[152] antiarthritic properties,[153] and inhibits TNF-α,[154,155] COX-2,[156] and lowers CRP levels.[157] In addition, guggul purifies the blood, supports the immune system, and aids comfortable movement of the joints. Avoid the use of guggul with synthetic hormone replacement therapy, and be cautious with anticoagulants, antiplatelet medications, thyroid medications and drug contraceptives. Dosage depends on the form used. The most common form is guggul resin extract, which is usually 375 to 750 mg twice daily. Less common are standardized supercitricidal CO_2 extracts (20 to 120 mg twice daily), and guggul leaf powder (210 mg twice daily).

Vitamin D is in fact a natural steroid hormone, not a true vitamin. Those with AS tend to have lower levels of vitamin D, which is associated with increased disease progression.[158,159] Vitamin D reduces proteins—IL-6 and TNF-α—that cause inflammation and binds to cell receptors that activate the MKP-1 gene—a gene that interferes with the inflammatory cascade.[160]

Some evidence even suggests that autoimmune disorders are associated with a dysfunction of vitamin D receptors (VDR) caused by pathogenic organisms, and that restoring VDR function can reverse autoimmune diseases and is involved in the autoinflammatory response.[161,162,163,164] Phenols found in essential oils are known to clean cell receptors and may be beneficial for VDR dysfunction.

High levels of vitamin D are required to affect serum vitamin D levels. Most individuals with AS will need to supplement with 3,000 to 8,000 IU of vitamin D3 (cholecalciferol) daily, preferably in softgel form and taken with some nuts or other source of healthy fat to improve bioavailability. Ideally serum levels should be checked before and during supplementation to ensure optimum levels are achieved—likely 50 ng/ml to 80 ng/ml.

Astaxanthin is a powerful antioxidant carotenoid with potent anti-inflammatory benefits. It is naturally found in some plants (like algae) and animals (especially seafood). It helps reduce CRP levels, modulates the immune response, helps eliminate bacteria, decreases oxidative stress and oxidative tissue damage, protects DNA from damage, and reduces systemic, eye, and gastric inflammation.[165,166,167,168,169,170] Studies have used dosages ranging from 2 to 8 mg, with 4 mg being the common dose available in dietary supplements.

Vitamin C is essential for collagen—a major component of connective tissues, and used by the body to restore joint elasticity—production. When ingested, vitamin C combines with lysine and proline to form procollagen—the precursor to the production of collagen. Some scientists propose that chronic deficiencies in vitamin C cause degeneration of spinal discs.[171] AS patients often have diminished levels of vitamin C, so supplementation is important to maintain healthy collagen.

Another benefit of vitamin C is its role in immune system activity. Vitamin C enhances natural killer cell activity and improves resilience to infectious diseases.[172] This is important for those who are taking medications for AS that are known to decrease the ability of the immune system to fight infections—adaluminab, many NSAIDs, etanercept, corticosteroids, and methotrexate. AS patients should take between 500 and 1,500 mg of vitamin C daily in divided doses. Vitamin C may increase blood estrogen levels when taken with drug contraceptives, could potentially interact with cholesterol medications and herbal remedies, and may interact with protease inhibitors.

Emerging evidence suggests that nicotinamide riboside (Niagen), which boosts production of the essential metabolite nicotinamide adenine dinucleotide (NAD^+),[173,174] may be useful for AS. NAD^+ regulates pathways involved in healthy aging, influences energy metabolism and mitochondrial production, and alters the immune response by converting destructive cells into protective cells. In other words, by increasing NAD+, nicotinamide riboside may reverse autoimmune and mitochondrial dysfunctions by converting cells that are damaging healthy tissue into cells that now protect and restore that tissue.[175,176] It may also boost energy levels. The typical dosage is 125 to 250 mg daily, although as much as 25 mg/kg of bodyweight has been used in studies.[177] It may interact with antidiabetic, ant seizure, high blood pressure, statins, and gout medications. It should be avoided with alcohol and nicotine patches.

ANKYLOSING SPONDYLITIS COMPLICATIONS

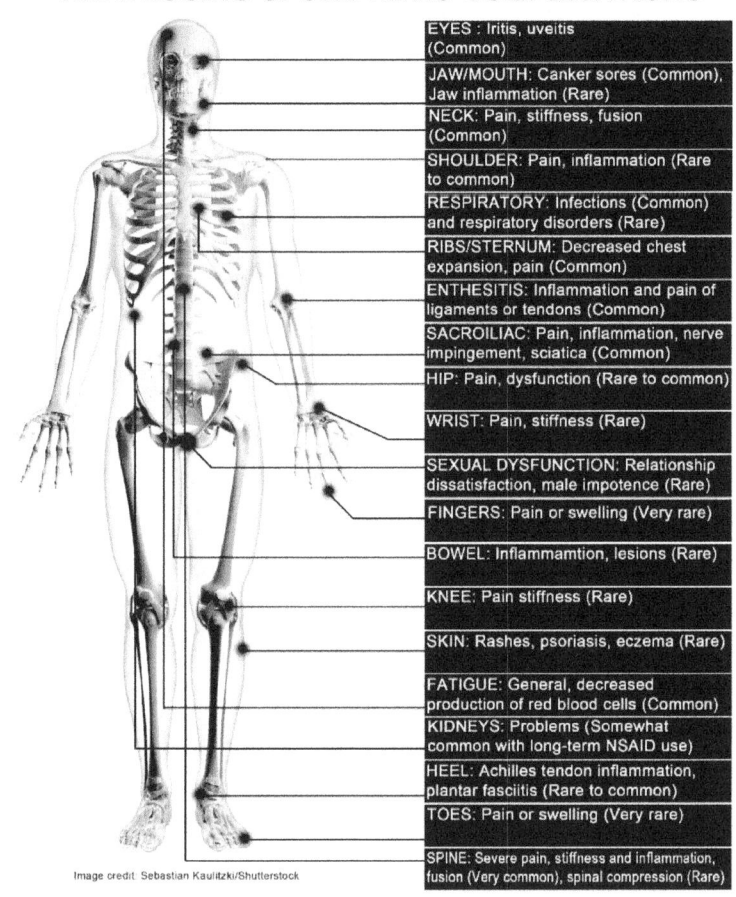

Area	Complications
EYES	Iritis, uveitis (Common)
JAW/MOUTH	Canker sores (Common), Jaw inflammation (Rare)
NECK	Pain, stiffness, fusion (Common)
SHOULDER	Pain, inflammation (Rare to common)
RESPIRATORY	Infections (Common) and respiratory disorders (Rare)
RIBS/STERNUM	Decreased chest expansion, pain (Common)
ENTHESITIS	Inflammation and pain of ligaments or tendons (Common)
SACROILIAC	Pain, inflammation, nerve impingement, sciatica (Common)
HIP	Pain, dysfunction (Rare to common)
WRIST	Pain, stiffness (Rare)
SEXUAL DYSFUNCTION	Relationship dissatisfaction, male impotence (Rare)
FINGERS	Pain or swelling (Very rare)
BOWEL	Inflammation, lesions (Rare)
KNEE	Pain stiffness (Rare)
SKIN	Rashes, psoriasis, eczema (Rare)
FATIGUE	General, decreased production of red blood cells (Common)
KIDNEYS	Problems (Somewhat common with long-term NSAID use)
HEEL	Achilles tendon inflammation, plantar fasciitis (Rare to common)
TOES	Pain or swelling (Very rare)
SPINE	Severe pain, stiffness and inflammation, fusion (Very common), spinal compression (Rare)

Image credit: Sebastian Kaulitzki/Shutterstock

Graphic Credit: Scott A. Johnson

Remedies for Complications of AS

As mentioned previously, AS is a highly adaptable and progressive disease that may affect many systems, organs, and areas of the body. The following are additional strategies to manage AS complications.

Peripheral joint pain and inflammation of the tendon and ligament insertion sites will largely be managed by the measures mentioned above. However, during flare-ups additional support may be required. During flare-ups consider applying Topricin®, Cristopher's Original Formulas® Complete Tissue & Bone Ointment, and Triflora®, and/or taking a homeopathic remedy. In addition, you may want to consider applying a drop or two of each of the following essential oils to the area of discomfort: lemongrass, marjoram, basil, and wintergreen, covered with DMSO cream.

Uveitis—inflammation of the middle layer of the eye, called the uvea—or iritis—inflammation of the iris of the eye—are fairly common among AS patients, with about one-third of patients experiencing them. Astaxanthin is able to cross the blood-retinal barrier and helps reduce eye inflammation, but the dosage may need to be increased to 8 mg during iritis or uveitis complications. I have also found that taking 7 drops copaiba, 5 drops frankincense and 3 drops cypress essential oil 1 to 3 times daily helps alleviate the eye inflammation. Also, I generally create a mixture of 2 drops each of basil, frankincense, lavender, copaiba, and helichrysum in 1 teaspoon of carrier oil (preferably grapeseed) and apply a couple drops of this mixture widely around the eye and behind the ears several times daily to obtain relief.

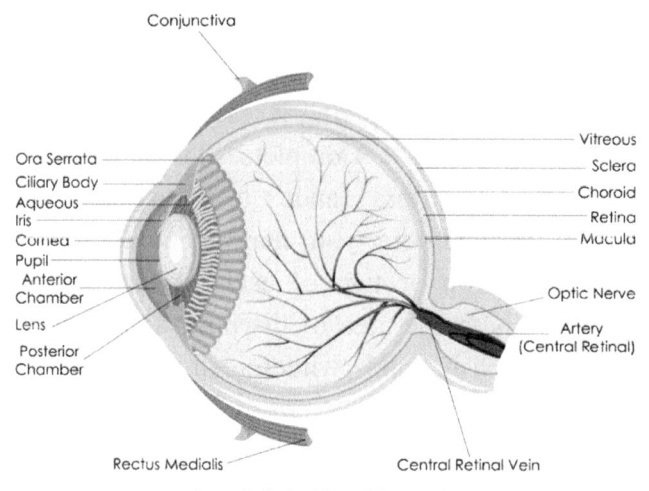

Image Credit: Stockshoppe/Shutterstock

Mouth ulcers or canker sores (aphthous ulcers) are largely caused by toothpastes that contain sulfur lauryl (or laureth) sulfate.[178] It is important that you use an SLS-free toothpaste to reduce the occurrence of sores—although it may take up to two months for a noticeable difference to occur after eliminating this irritating substance from your mouth. Taking a DGL tablet three times daily may help reduce the severity and duration of sores.[179,180] It may also be useful to apply one drop of peppermint, clove, lemon or tea tree oil to the ulcer (rotating which essential oil you use) several times daily.

AS and inflammatory bowel diseases (IBD)—Crohn's, ulcerative colitis—are occasionally seen together, with up to 10 percent of AS patients experiencing an inflammatory bowel disease.[181] A significant challenge among those who have AS and

IBD concurrently, is that the use of NSAIDs may exacerbate or trigger IBD. Long-term NSAID use may cause bowel inflammation among those who are prone to it, or cause IBD flare-ups.[182]

One of the most important things you can do to reduce the occurrence of bowel diseases and lesions is to eat a high-fiber, predominantly plant-based diet. Probiotics are also critical to support digestion and elimination and reduce intestinal inflammation. Enteric-coated peppermint capsules—to ensure the peppermint makes it to the intestines rather than irritating the esophagus—have demonstrated significant benefits for inflammatory bowel diseases.[183] DGL, slippery elm (800 mg two to three times daily),[184] and glutamine (2 to 4 g every four hours)[185] may all promote the healing of lesions and irritated tissues in the gastrointestinal tract, as well as reduce intestinal inflammation. Lastly, drinking aloe vera juice (about 3.5 ounces of a 50% solution twice daily) may reduce intestinal inflammation.[186]

Enteric-coated peppermint may interfere with the metabolism of several medications. It is also theoretically possible that slippery elm could reduce intestinal absorption of some drugs. Glutamine should be used cautiously if you are taking anticonvulsants or while undergoing chemotherapy. Aloe vera should not be taken with digoxin, anticoagulants, or stimulant laxatives, and may interfere with intestinal absorption of some medications.

Another important targeted nutrient that helps repair intestinal permeability that is foundational to autoinflammatory conditions is quercetin. Research has determined that quercetin improves the intestinal barrier and reduces intestinal inflammation by influencing the production of tight junction proteins.[187,188] The typical dosage of quercetin is 500 mg twice daily. Quercetin may interact with specific antibiotics, blood thinners, and high blood pressure medications.

Other nutrients that have also demonstrated the ability to improve the intestinal barrier are naringenin,[189] fucoidan,[190] and glutamine.[191,192] Naringenin is usually combined with other bioflavonoids (flavonones). Fucoidan supplements usually supply a dose of 80 and 300 mg twice daily. It may interact with blood thinners. A maintenance dosage of glutamine may be 2,000 mg one to three times daily.

Enthesitis is fairly common in AS patients, particularly of the Achilles tendon and plantar fascia calcaneal insertions. However, inflammation can occur anywhere a tendon, ligament, joint capsule, or fascia attaches to bone. For this type of pain I have found *arnica montana* to be beneficial. Essential oils can also provide great relief. Applying a combination of wintergreen, lemongrass, marjoram, cypress, and basil to the affected area can be very soothing. Wintergreen may interact with aspirin and should not be used by children under age 12, or those who are pregnant or nursing. It is best to apply these essential oils about four hours after taking any medications to reduce the likelihood of an unintended interaction.

Applying ice packs to the affected area for 20 minutes at a time, three times daily is also helpful for enthesitis. For Achilles enthesitis, perform straight knee and bent knee calf raises three times per day. To perform straight knee calf raises, stand on a firm floor with your legs straight and feet flat. Slowly raise your heels until you are on your tip toes and hold for three seconds before dropping back to flat feet. To perform bent knee calf raises begin with your feet flat on the ground and bend your knees slightly. Straighten your knees as you raise on you tip toes and hold for three seconds before returning to the starting position. Perform 15 repetitions with the knee straight and 15 with the knee bent.

The risk of adverse cardiovascular disorders—including aortic insufficiency, cardiomyopathy, myocarditis that causes conduction disturbances, left ventricular dysfunction, and atherosclerosis[193,194,195,196]—is possible with AS. A well-established heart nutrient is the coenzyme Q10 (CoQ10), and research suggests CoQ10 deficiencies are associated with aortic insufficiencies. In addition, CoQ10 improves left ventricular function, improves cardiomyopathy, protects against viral myocarditis, and improves endothelial function—endothelial dysfunction is linked to atherosclerosis.[197,198,199,200,201] The active form of CoQ10, ubiquinol, is the preferred and most bioavailable form of CoQ10. Ubiquinol is an unstable nutrient and should be stabilized, or it will oxidize to its less active form ubiquinone. Therapeutic dosages range from 50 to 100 mg three times per day, and up to 3,000 mg per day. A preventive dose may be 50 to 100 mg daily. CoQ10 may interact with anticoagulant, chemotherapy, and antihypertensive drugs.

Another lesser-known, but highly effective heart nutrient is the Indian gooseberry (also called amla, amalki, amlaki, and *Phyllanthus embillica*). Research suggests that Indian Gooseberry improves cholesterol profiles and endothelial function as effectively as the drug atorvastatin, causes cardiovascular adaptations that result in greater heart injury protection, protects against viral myocarditis, and prevents drug-induced heart toxicity—better than other tested antioxidants.[202,203,204,205,206] Dosages range from 250 to 1,000 mg twice daily.

Essential oils can profoundly influence the cardiovascular system by helping to normalize blood pressure, reduce inflammation (myocarditis), and support normal cholesterol levels. Some essential oils to consider applying over the heart include copaiba, ylang ylang, helichrysum, marjoram, and lavender.

The human body forms about 2 million red blood cells (erythrocytes) every second, making them the most abundant cells in the human body. A number of vitamins and minerals are necessary to form red blood cells including iron, copper, and vitamins A, folate (B9), B12, B6, and E. If you are taking an optimum potency multi-nutrient you should get sufficient quantities of these nutrients to support normal red blood cell production.

Lipids known as alkyglycerols are known to increase red blood cell production in animals.[207,208] Alkyglycerols are abundantly found in shark liver oil. Most supplements provide 500 to 1,000 mg of shark liver oil daily. Lemon essential oil is also believed to support red blood cell production. This may be due to the high limonene content of citrus oils, which is known to stimulate the production of GSH—an erythrocyte protecting antioxidant. Erythrocytes are highly susceptible to oxidative damage and increasing GSH levels may preserve them from destruction.[209] Five to 10 drops of lemon essential oil daily in a capsule may be supportive of normal red blood cell turnover—the replacement of old red blood cells with newly produced ones (red blood cells normally have a lifespan of 120 days).

Chronic inflammation of the spine may result in scar tissue buildup that gradually traps nerve roots in the lower spine—a condition known as sciatica. Sciatica is pain that radiates from your lower back through your hips and down the buttocks and leg. It occurs when the sciatic nerve is irritated, pinched, or compressed due to a ruptured disc, injury, narrowing of the spinal canal, or overgrowth of bone near the sacroiliac joint.

Acupressure is useful in releasing pressure on the nerves that cause sciatic pain. It is possible to have another person apply pressure to relieve sciatic pain as follows. Have another person apply pressure to acupressure point GB 30 (pictured above), which can be found in the side of the buttocks by locating approximately the middle of the sacrum, and then moving out two-thirds of the way toward the hip. Apply firm pressure to this point (left or right side one at a time) with your thumb for about 30 seconds, then release. Repeat this process until pain is relieved. Then repeat the entire process on the other side.

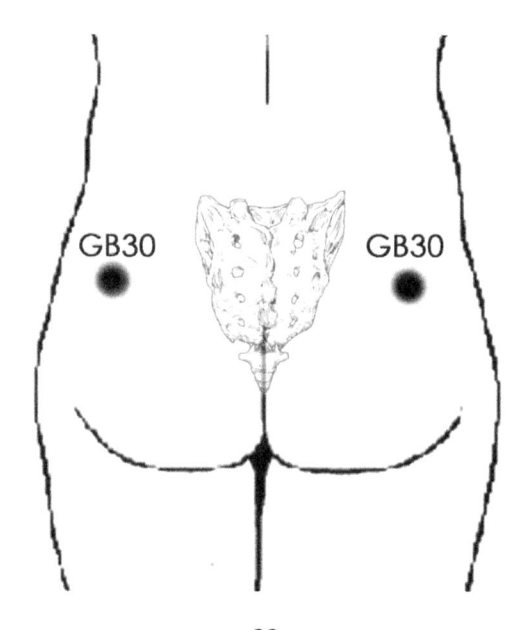

Exercises can also be performed to alleviate pressure on the sciatic nerve and increase range of motion in the sacroiliac joint.

Knee to Chest Stretch: Lay flat on your back with your legs bent and feet on the floor approximately one and a half feet from your buttocks. Slowly bring one knee to your chest, pumping the leg gently a few times at the top of the range of motion, then lower the leg to the original position. Repeat the exercise with the other leg, completing 10 repetitions with each leg.

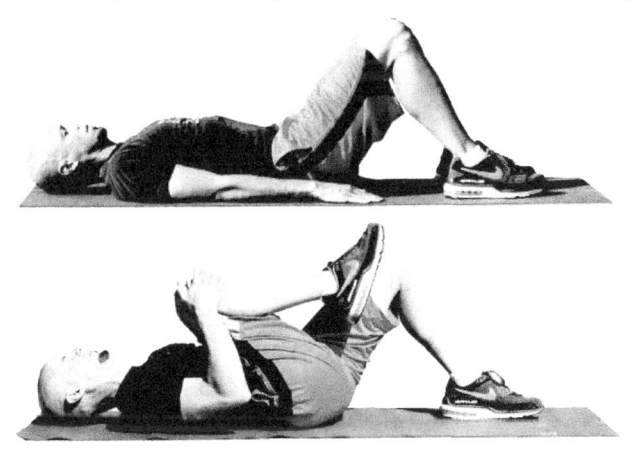

Back Extensions: Lie flat on your stomach with your forearms flat on the ground and palms facing down, so that your elbows are about midway down your chest. Push up, supporting your upper body with your forearms and elbows until your back reaches about a 45-degree angle from the floor. Lengthen your spine, keeping your shoulders back and neck long, and keeping your pelvis in contact with the floor. Hold this position for about 10 seconds then slowly lower back to the floor. Repeat this exercise 10 times, gradually working to hold the position for 30 seconds.

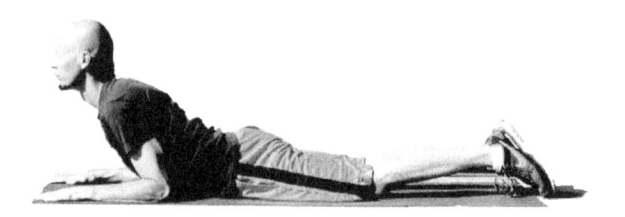

Chair Leg Raises: Sit on a chair or other sturdy surface with your legs bent and feet touching the floor. Slowly raise one leg until it is parallel with the chair seat, while simultaneously raising your head to look up at the ceiling. Hold for five seconds and repeat the exercise 10 times. Then complete the exercise with the other leg 10 times.

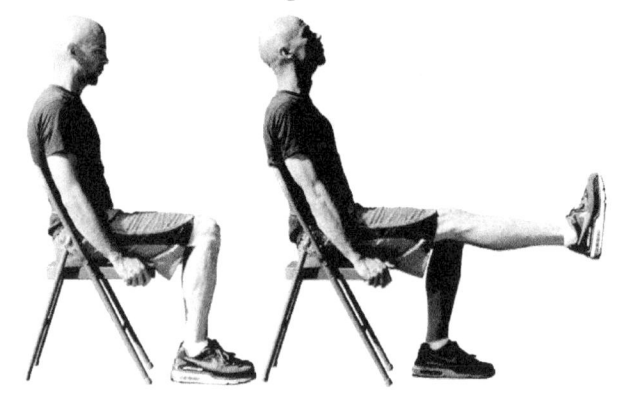

Sitting Hip Stretch: Sit on the floor with the soles of your feet together about one foot from your groin, and your knees lowered to the floor as far as possible. Similar to a groin stretch, grab your feet and slowly bend your upper body forward while maintaining a straight spine until you feel a gentle stretch in your hip joints. Hold the pose for 20 to 30 seconds and then relax. Repeat the exercise three times.

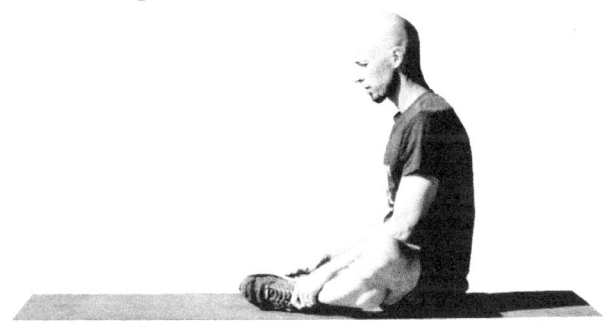

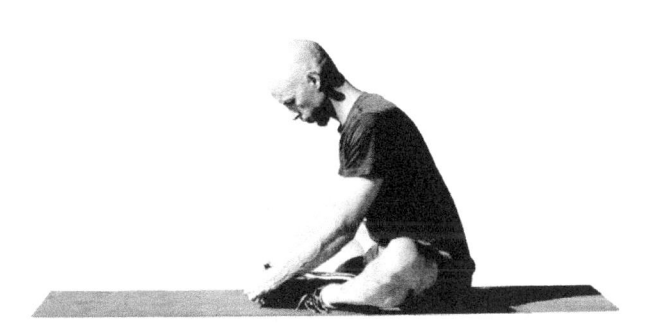

Sciatic Hamstring Stretch: Lie on your back with your knees bent and feet flat on the floor hip-width apart and about one foot from your buttocks. Raise one leg up towards your chest while holding underneath your hamstring with both hands. Flex your toes towards your head and straighten the leg completely (if possible). Hold for 20 to 30 seconds and then return to the starting position. Repeat the exercise for the other leg. And repeat the exercise for each leg three times total. Only stretch as far as comfortable and stop if you feel any pain, tingling, or numbness with all but the Chair Leg Raises, which may increase sciatica symptoms during the stretch.

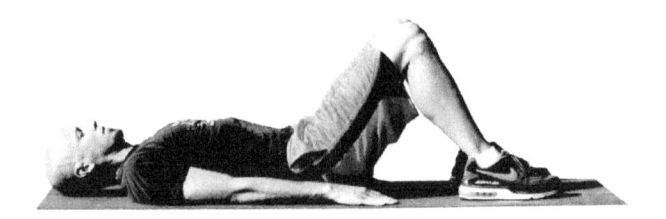

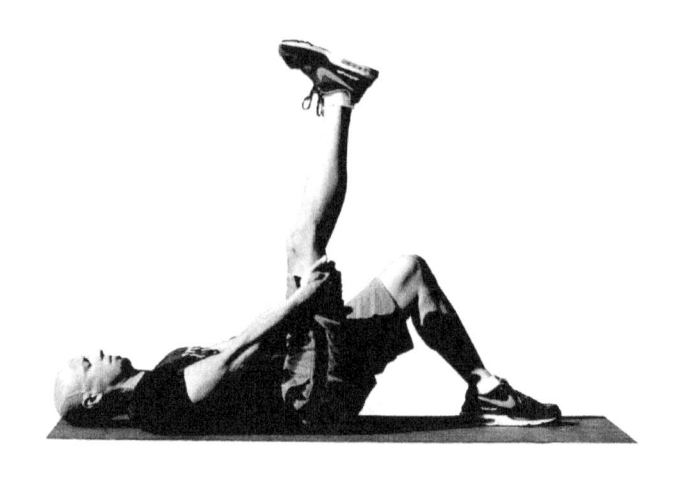

In addition, chronic inflammation and attacks on the joints in the neck can cause damage to the cervical portion of the spine. This damage causes a narrowing of the vertebral column, which compresses the spinal cord, leading to pain, numbness, and weakness—called cervical myelopathy. Glucosamine and chondroitin can help preserve the cartilage between each vertebra, as can the application of Cristopher's Original Formulas® Complete Tissue & Bone Ointment. This is the most practical way to mitigate this complication. You may also need to see a physical therapist to manage cervical myelopathy (exercises, mobilization, ultrasound, electrical stimulation).

Though less common than other AS complications, skin rashes may occur in conjunction with AS. They often appear as red, scaly, patchy rashes similar to psoriasis. One of the best ways to manage rashes is to keep the area moist with a hypoallergenic, fragrance-free lotion. In addition, several homeopathic creams provide relief. Some that I have found to work well include:
- Florasone® — contains cardiospermum, which possesses natural cortisone-like properties and relieves rashes, itching, and inflammation.
- Califlora® — a homeopathic calendula gel that relieves chapped and irritated skin.
- Psoriaflora® — contains *Berberis aquifolium*, a homeopathic remedy for dry scaly skin.

In addition to topical ointments, it is important to take additional probiotics (four times daily) and possibly increase the amount of MSM you are taking to 2,500 mg four times daily when experiencing skin rashes.

Bladder dysfunction, such as incontinence, is rare with AS, but may occur occasionally. If you experience bladder problems, the primary action you should take is to start performing Kegel exercises daily. These are performed by contracting the same muscles (pelvic muscles) that stop urination. The easiest way to identify these muscles is to stop urine flow midstream. Men can also identify these muscles by observing this muscle contraction in the mirror. When the muscle is contracted a man's penis will move closer to his belly and his testicles will rise. The muscles used to stop urine flow are the same muscles you want to strengthen to reduce incontinence.

To perform Kegel exercises, empty your bladder, then lie on you back. Tighten your pelvic muscles and hold this contraction for 5 to 10 seconds. Rest for 10 seconds then repeat the tightening procedure. Do this five times and repeat the five repetitions three to five times per day. For men, Kegel exercises may also decrease symptoms of premature ejaculation.

Magnesium and vitamin D are important nutrients for bladder function, and you should get enough of them through diet and your supplementation plan (optimum multi-nutrient). Essential oils may also be of benefit. Apply three to five drops of cypress over the bladder area two to four times daily. For additional support, apply one drop each of frankincense and cedarwood diluted in a carrier oil to the area between the anus and vagina/scrotum.

Sexual dysfunction is another uncommon complication of AS in both men and women. However, women with AS report their dissatisfaction as sexual relationship difficulties, whereas men with AS may experience a functional issue—erectile dysfunction (ED)—during sexual intercourse. Sexual dysfunction—and the relationship dissatisfaction for that matter—may effectively be due to the anxiety and stress of maintaining normal sexual relations when pain, stiffness, and the movements of sexual intercourse may aggravate AS symptoms. All of the measures that have been mentioned throughout this book will help maintain normal sexual performance and enjoyment for both sexes. If men do experience ED, natural remedies may improve the ability to maintain a satisfactory erection.

One of the most commonly recommended herbal remedies for ED is yohimbee, or its active ingredient yohimbine. But, both yohimbee and yohimbine tend to have serious side effects—irregular heartbeat, confusion, dizziness, anxiety, tremors, and headache—so they should be used only as an absolute last resort.

A better option is Panax ginseng, which research suggests improves male sexual performance and erectile function.[210,211] Typical dosages range from 600 to 900 mg three times daily. Panax ginseng should not be taken with alcohol or caffeine, and may interact with antidiabetic, anticoagulant, antiplatelet, immunosuppressant, antidepressant, and blood thinning drugs.

L-arginine may also help as it relaxes blood vessels—through increased nitric oxide production—to help produce and maintain an erection. Studies have used from 1.7 to 5 grams daily for ED—some combined with pycnogenol.[212,213] L-arginine should not be used with antihypertensive or nitrate medications and may also interact with ED drugs (Viagra®, Cialis®).

A number of respiratory conditions may develop during the course of AS, including common fungal and mycobacterial infections.[214] It is thought that respiratory conditions affect a little more than half of AS patients, but the conditions are often mild and asymptomatic.[215] Serious respiratory disorders are rare.

Ginger essential oil is not often thought of as a respiratory-supporting remedy, but research suggests that it reduces inflammation of the airway and triggers bronchodilation[216]—widening of the bronchi and bronchioles, therefore increasing airflow to the lungs. The scientists attributed the bronchodilatory action of ginger essential oil to its citral content. If this finding is true, myrtle and lemongrass (*Cymbopogon citratus*)—both near 90 percent citral content would likely produce similar effects.

Myrtle essential oil is commonly used to support the respiratory system and provides a powerful relaxant effect to this system. Research suggests that myrtle reduces spasms, opens the airways through bronchodilation, and improves blood flow to the lungs through vasodilation[217]—the widening of blood vessels.

Lemongrass essential oil possesses anti-inflammatory, antibacterial, antiviral, anti-amoebic, anti-parasitic, antimycobacterial, and antifungal properties that make it useful for a variety of respiratory infections. It has also demonstrated the ability to protect lung cells from DNA damage and prevent the spread of lung cancer.[218,219]

Eucalyptus essential oil is another oil traditionally used for a variety of respiratory complaints. Evidence suggests that the eucalyptus species can relax the smooth muscle of the airways, reduce lung inflammation, and prevent the spread of lung cancer carcinomas.[220,221,222]

To support respiratory health, or to eliminate a respiratory infection, apply a few drops of myrtle, ginger, lemongrass, eucalyptus, and pine (helps expel mucous from the airways) essential oils in a carrier oil to the upper back and chest one to four times daily. It may also be useful to diffuse or steam inhale one or more of the above oils.

Sleep apnea is considered a respiratory disorder, and is characterized by frequent interruptions or disruptions of breathing during sleep. Excess weight, high blood pressure, and alcohol consumption are all contributing factors in sleep apnea and should be addressed. In addition, some report improvement by applying one to three drops of thyme and/or black spruce essential oil on the bottoms of each big toe and bottoms of the feet each night before retiring to bed.

If fatigue is an issue, DGL isn't the only remedy that may give you a much needed pick-me-up. Simply inhaling peppermint, rosemary, and basil essential oils may provide a mental and physical boost. These essential oils may also help improve poor concentration and memory often reported among AS patients. In addition, an optimum potency B-complex vitamin supports your body's ability to produce energy.

Another option is cordyceps, which has even been used by Olympic athletes to improve energy levels, athletic performance, and stamina. It appears to provide broad benefits to a number of body systems and organs including immune, endocrine, cardiovascular, respiratory, nervous, sexual, and the kidney and liver.[223,224] Animal studies suggest that cordyceps enhances endurance, reduces blood lactic acid levels, and activates muscle metabolic regulators.[225,226] A human study with older adults showed that cordyceps improved athletic performance, respiratory capacity, and muscle endurance.[227] The usual dosage of fermented cordyceps is 3,000 mg daily. It is possible that cordyceps could interfere with immunosuppressive medications due to its immunostimulant activity.

Other possible anti-fatigue nutrients include:
- Siberian ginseng—used for centuries to reduce mental and physical fatigue and enhance performance, Siberian ginseng is an adaptogen, meaning it may support the body's ability to adapt to both physical and mental stress. Up to 1,200 mg of Siberian ginseng is taken daily to enhance energy levels and improve athletic performance. It should not be taken with alcohol and may interact with anticoagulant, antiplatelet, antidiabetic, CNS depressant, cardiac, and mood-stabilizing medications.
- D-ribose—increases the levels and availability of ATP (adenosine triphosphate), which is essential for the production of energy, and may reduce post-exercise fatigue.
- Gynostemma (also called jiaogulan)—thought to produce cellular energy molecules ATP and creatine phosphate. Gynostemma may also modulate the immune system.[228] The typical dose of gynostemma extract is 250 to 500 mg twice daily. It may interact with anticoagulant, antiplatelet, and immunosuppressive drugs.

AS SUPPLEMENT PLAN
(PRIMARY MANAGEMENT)

Supplement	Dosage
Multi-nutrient	Optimum levels of vitamins, minerals and other nutrients
Marine Omega-3s	Providing 500 mg each of DHA and EPA
Probiotic	8 billion organisms once daily; four times daily with rashes. (Look for *Lactobacillus GG, L. casei, L. reuteri, L. rhamnosus RC-14,* and *L. rhamnosus GR1)*
Turmeric/Curcumin	500 to 1,000 mg twice daily
Ginger	170 to 255 mg three times daily
MSM	500 mg three times daily
	2,500 mg four times daily for skin rashes
Glucosamine	500 mg three times daily
Chondroitin	400 mg three times daily
Boswellia Serrata Extract	300 to 500 mg three times daily
Quercetin	500 mg twice daily
Astaxanthin	4 mg daily
Vitamin C	500 mg three times daily
Vitamin D	3,000 to 8,000 IU daily
Nicotinamide Ribose	125 to 250 mg daily

AS NECESSARY OR ROTATE IN PLAN

Supplement	Dosage
Proteolytic Enzymes	According to supplement label
Guggul Resin Extract	375 to 750 mg twice daily
DGL	380 to 400 mg up to three times daily
Rhus toxicodendron	30C potency, take as described on the supplement label
Kali carbonicum	30C potency, take as described in the label
Slippery Elm	800 mg two to three times daily
Glutamine	2 to 4 g every four waking hours for the first two to three weeks then 2 g one to three times daily as a maintenance dose
Naringenin	According to supplement label
Fucoidan	80 to 300 mg twice daily
Aloe vera (50% solution)	3.5 ounces twice daily
Enteric-coated peppermint	Two 180 to 225 mg capsules daily
CoQ10 (ubiquinol)	Preventive: 50 to 100 mg daily Therapeutic: Up to 3,000 mg daily in divided doses
Indian Gooseberry	250 to 1,000 mg twice daily
Panax Ginseng	600 to 900 mg three times daily
L-arginine	1.7 to 5 g daily
Cordyceps	Up to 3,000 mg daily
Siberian Ginseng	Up to 1,200 mg daily
Gynostemma	25 to 500 mg twice daily

Lifestyle Considerations and Ankylosing Spondylitis

Before parting, there are a few additional tips to help you better manage AS.

Getting a good night's rest can be a challenge when you experience the pain and discomfort of AS, but it is critical to your management plan. Sleep is a two-edged sword for people with AS because lack of movement makes the pain and stiffness worse, but inadequate sleep can lead to an increase in morning stiffness, overall pain, anxiety, depression, and general malaise.[229,230] This can quickly become a vicious cycle that causes flare ups. Some tips to improve sleep quality include:
- Give yourself some time to wind down and relax prior to going to bed.
- Do some light spine articulation exercises before going to bed.
- Make sure your room is completely dark to support sleep.
- Make your bedroom as quiet as possible.
- Reserve your bed for sleep and intimacy—not television watching or reading.
- Keep your sleep routine as consistent as possible.

- Sleep on your back to maintain proper posture while sleeping.

While also related to sleep, your pillow and mattress are so important they deserve more than just a bullet point. I experienced frequent neck pain and headaches until I switched to an orthopedic pillow that supported my neck in the correct anatomical position. These pillows are readily available and worth the investment for the significant improvement in sleep quality and duration. Choose a mattress that is firm and helps support the natural "S-curve" of your spine while on your back—which is the best position to sleep in—and keeps it straight while lying on your side.

Practicing good posture will help prevent spine pain and reduce the pronounced curvature of the spine that may occur gradually with AS. Whether sitting or standing, strive to keep your chin up and your head in line with your spine. Think of it this way; your spine is like a stack of blocks that must support a larger block (your head) on top. In order to keep the tower of blocks sturdy enough to support the larger block you must keep your spine (the tower of blocks) straight and your head (the larger block on top) directly over the spine to prevent spillage.

One way to check your posture is against a wall. If your feet are four inches from the wall, your buttocks and shoulders should be touching or very close to touching the wall. Be mindful of slouching when sitting. It is natural for us to want to slouch—and may even be more comfortable, but remember a straight back keeps your head properly supported and also decreases spinal pain.

Ergonomics are important in virtually every daily activity you participate in, both at home and at work. Adjust desk heights and sit in an appropriate chair—hard-backed rather than soft chairs or sofas—that provides support for the spine. If you sit at a desk for extended periods, stand up and stretch at least every 30 minutes. Corsets and braces are generally unnecessary, ineffective, and not recommended for people with AS.

Many newer vehicles have a lumbar support built into the seat. Lumbar support while driving can reduce pain and stiffness and support the natural "S-curve" of the spine. If your vehicle does not come equipped with lumbar support, purchase a lumbar support cushion. Frequent stops to stretch on a long drive will also reduce pain and stiffness.

A simple way to release tension and relieve pressure on the spine and other parts of the body is an Alexander Technique called constructive rest. To do this lie flat on your back with support under your head and your feet resting parallel on a chair; or with a pillow or roll under your knees so your feet are flat on the ground. It may also be done with only your heels touching the ground. Remain in this position for about 20 minutes daily.

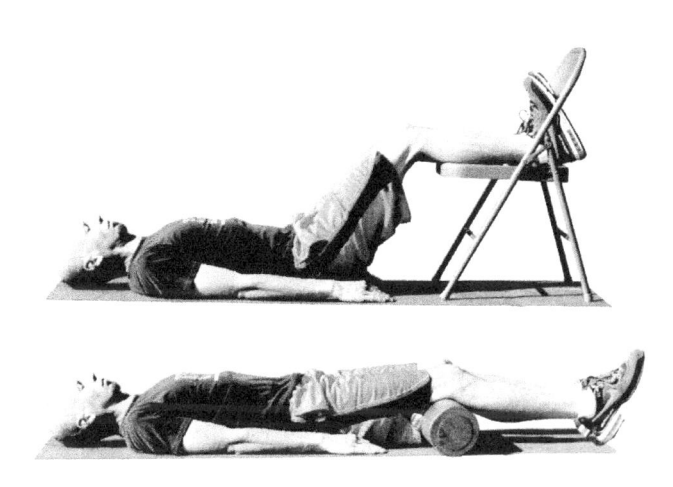

Heat and cold applications may decrease pain and stiffness, particularly if you use some heat to warm your muscles before exercise. Heat can be applied in a bath, shower, or hot tub, or with a heating pad. To enhance the benefits of a hot bath, add a cup of Epsom salts with a few drops of lavender and or ginger essential oil in the salts. Be aware that applying heat too often may actually increase inflammation to the area of application. Indeed, one small study found that heat therapy triggers the inflammatory process in individuals with AS.[231]

If an area is significantly inflamed or swollen, ice is a better option and will help decrease the localized inflammation. In fact, whole-body cryotherapy (WBC) is commonly used to relieve the pain and inflammation associated with AS and other chronic inflammatory conditions.[232] WBC is regularly used by athletes to enhance recovery times and involves exposure to extremely cold temperatures—from 170 to more than 200 degrees Fahrenheit below zero—in a refrigerator-like device for two to three minutes. The person receiving WBC usually wears a bathing suit or shorts, gloves, dry socks, and a headband to protect the ears from the damaging effects of the extreme temperatures.

Pilot studies investigating the effects of WBC on inflammatory rheumatic diseases have been promising, demonstrating reductions in pain—for about 90 minutes following treatment—and disease activity, as well as improvements in functionality.[233,234] One study determined that WBC produces significant improvements in lumbar and thoracic spinal mobility.[235]

Daily deep breathing exercises are imperative to maintain respiratory health and optimum chest wall expansion capabilities. The chest constricting nature of AS can make taking a deep breath very difficult, but deep breathing helps prevent stiffening and fusion of the ribs and maintains the flexibility of the chest wall, protecting your ability to inhale deeply.

To perform deep breathing exercises, sit at the front of a sturdy chair with your feet on the floor about hip distance apart and your back straight. Your arms should rest on your upper legs with your hands on your knees. Raise your hands straight in front of you and over your head—like you are signaling a touchdown, except your palms are facing forward—while taking a deep inhalation through your nostrils.

The inhalation should expand your abdomen as well as your chest. Exhale very slowly through your nose as you slowly lower your arms to the starting position. Repeat for 10 to 20 breaths twice daily. To enhance this activity, diffuse or inhale a respiratory supporting essential oil like peppermint, eucalyptus, or myrtle while performing deep breathing exercises.

No resource would be complete without discussing the mood disturbances that may occur with AS—anxiety, depression, and stress—and how they affect disease progression. It is clear that those with AS who report significant anxiety or depression also frequently experience worse symptoms, decreased quality of life, accelerated disease activity, and poorer general well-being.[236,237,238,239] Therefore, it is very important to manage stress, anxious feelings, and depressive symptoms as much as possible. Consider the following suggestions:

- Laughter releases endorphins and other chemicals that can enhance mood and increase pain tolerance levels. Enjoy some laughter every day.
- Citrus essential oils are strongly uplifting. If you need help with lingering sadness, consider inhaling a citrus essential oil or apply a few drops on your feet three times each day.
- St. John's Wort, SAMe, and 5-HTP are also useful in managing mild to moderate depression. These natural options should not

be taken with antidepressant medications. Check with your doctor or pharmacist for interactions and contraindications for each of these remedies.
- Kava kava, chamomile tea, L-theanine, and lemon balm may help relieve anxious feelings. Consult a qualified professional before taking these natural remedies.
- Perform deep breathing exercises for a few minutes every day.
- Consider lavender and German chamomile essential oils to relieve stress. Both lavender and German chamomile are known to help reduce cortisol levels, thus affecting stress levels by altering body biochemistry.[240,241] These can be inhaled, applied on the wrists, or massaged on the shoulders and back for stress relief.

Lastly, join a support group or web forum to learn from and share with others with AS. Participating in a support group helps you understand that you are not alone, and that others are experiencing many of the same things you are. A support group gives you a network of people that understand you, know AS and its myriad symptoms, and have experience with several treatment options, allowing you access to a panel of knowledgeable people to discuss and compare symptoms, treatments, and other useful management strategies with. Search the Internet for groups near you, or online groups that you are interested in joining. But remember, this group doesn't need to be at a physical location, nor near your home—there are many groups for you to join on the Internet and even on Facebook.

Conclusion

By now you should have a better understanding of AS and what you can do to proactively manage it, so that you can enjoy a happier and healthier life. Don't be overwhelmed with everything that is shared in this book, take things one step at a time. It is meant to be comprehensive and to provide a variety of strategies so that each person can experiment with what works best for him or her and rotate therapies to keep AS on its toes.

Start by incorporating a few strategies and monitor how it affects you. Keep a journal of foods you eat, supplements you take, physical activity you participate in, etc., to help you identify triggers and things that help. Don't give up if you don't see immediate results. Your results will vary based on disease progression, how long you have had AS, and your current state of health. Some remedies may take weeks to produce results. Keep trying and maintain a "can do" attitude. You can beat AS because anything is possible.

AS is not a death sentence and can be managed well by incorporating the recommendations in this book. I am proof of that—approaching a decade of beating AS naturally (as of this writing). I wish you abundant success and a happy, healthy, and fulfilling life.

About the Author:

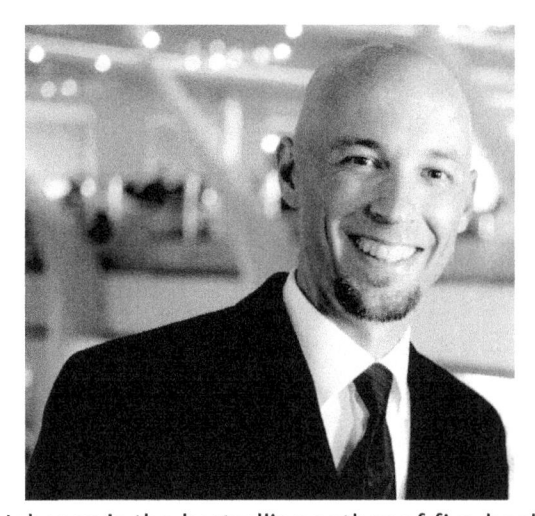

Scott Johnson is the bestselling author of five books and more than 250 articles featured in online and print publications. He holds a doctorate in naturopathy and is a board certified Alternative Medical Practitioner (AMP) and Certified Clinical Master Aromatherapist (CCMA). His evidence-based approach to natural healing, experience conducting medical research, and ability to unite the art of natural healing with science, makes him a leading expert in natural medicine. Scott draws on his wealth of experience and diverse educational background as he travels the globe to share the secrets of natural healing with those who seek greater wellness.

Connect with Scott:

FACEBOOK:
https://www.facebook.com/AuthorScottAJohnson
TWITTER:
https://twitter.com/DocScottJohnson

REFERENCES

[1] Ambarus C, Yeremenko N, Tak P, et al. Pathogenesis of spondyloarthritis: autoimmune or autoinflammatory? *Urr Opin Rheumatol.* 2012 Jul;24(4):351-8.

[2] Seo MR, Baek HL, Yoon HH, et al. Delayed diagnosis is linked to worse outcomes and unfavourable treatment responses in patient with axial spondyloarthritis. *Clin Rheumatol.* 2014 Sep 5. [Epub ahead of print]

[3] Lee W, Reveille J, Davis Jr, J, et al. Are there gender differences in severity of ankylosing spondylitis? Results from the PSOAS cohort. *Ann Rheum Dis.* 2007;66:633-38.

[4] Van der Horst-Bruinsma IE, Zack DJ, Szumski A, et al. Female patients with ankylosing spondylitis: analysis of the impact of gender across treatment studies. *Ann Rheum Dis.* 2013 Jul;72(7):1221-24.

[5] Momeni M, Taylor N, Tehrani M. Cardiopulmonary manifestations of ankylosing spondylitis. *Int J Rheumatol.* 2011;2011:728471.

[6] Yildirir A, Aksoyek S, Calguneri M, et al. QT dispersion as a predictor of arrhythmic events in patients with ankylosing spondylitis. *Rheumatology.* 2000;39(8):875-79.

[7] Carter ET, McKenna CH, Brian DD, et al. Epidemiology of ankylosing spondylitis in Rochester, Minnesota, 1935-1973. *Arthritis Rheum.* 1979;22:365-70.

[8] Helmick C, Felson D, Lawrence R, et al. Estimates of the prevalence of arthritis and other rheumatic conditions in the United States. Part 1. *Arthritis Rheum.* 2008 Jan;58(1):15-25.

[9] Sheehan N. The ramification of HLA-B27. *J R Soc Med.* 2004 Jan;97(1):1-14.

[10] Roberts R, Wallace M, Jones G, et al. Prevalence of HLA-B27 in the New Zealand population: effect of age and ethnicity. *Arthritis Res Ther.* 2013 Oct;15(5):R158.

[11] Garcia-Medel N, Sanz-Bravo A, Alvarez-Navarro C, et al. Peptide handling by HLA-B27 subtypes influences their biological behavior, association with ankylosing spondylitis and susceptibility to ERAP1. *Mol Cell Proteomics.* 2014 Sep 3. [Epub ahead of print]

[12] Keidel S, Chen L, Pointon J, et al. ERAP1 and ankylosing spondylitis. *Curr Opin Immunol.* 2013 Feb;25(1):97-102.

[13] Martin-Esteban A, Gomez-Molina P, Sanz-Bravo, et al. Combined effects of ankylosing spondylitis-associated ERAP1 polymorphisms outside the catalytic and peptide-binding sites on the processing of natural HLA-B27 lignands. *J Biol Chem.* 2014 Feb;289(7):3978-90.

[14] Zhang Z, Dai D, Yu K, et al. Association of HLA-B27 and ERAP1 with ankylosing spondylitis susceptibility in Beijing Han Chinese. *Tiss Antigens.* 2014 May;83(5):324-29.

[15] Costello ME, Elewaut D, Kenna TJ, et al. Microbes, the gut and ankylosing spondylitis. *Arthritis Res Ther.* 2013;15(3):214.

[16] Rashid T, Ebringer A. Gut-mediated and HLA-B27-associated arthritis: An emphasis on ankylosing spondylitis and Crohn's disease with a proposal for the use of new treatment. *Discov Med.* 2011 Sep;12(64):187-94.

[17] Rashid T, Wilson C, Ebringer A. The link between ankylosing spondylitis, Crohn's disease, Klebsiella, and starch consumption. *Clin Dev Immunology.* 2013:2013:872632.

[18] Madhavan R, Porkodi R, Rajendran CP, et al. IgM, IgG, and IgA response to enterobacteria in patients with ankylosing spondylitis in southern India. *Ann N Y Acad Sci.* 2002 Apr;958:408-11.

[19] Pereira DF, Pinheiro MM, Silva PF, et al. Influence of TNF-α blockers on the oral prevalence of opportunistic microorganisms in ankylosing spondylitis, *Clin Exp Rheumatol.* 2012 Sep-Oct;30(5):679-85.

[20] Syrbe U, Scheer R, Wu P, et al. Differential synovial Th1 cell reactivity towards Escherichia coli antigens in patients with ankylosing spondylitis and rheumatoid arthritis. *Ann Rheum Dis.* 2012 Sep;71(9):1573-76.

[21] Feng XG, Xu XJ, Lin YY, et al. Recent Chlamydia pneumoniae infection is highly associated with active ankylosing spondylitis in a Chinese cohort. *Scand J Rheumatol.* 211;40(4):289-91.

[22] Rosenbaum JT, Davey MP. Time for a gut check: evidence for the hypothesis that HLA-B27 predisposes to ankylosing spondylitis by altering the microbiome. *Arthritis Rheum.* 2011 Nov;63(11):3195-98.

[23] Cusick MF, Libbey JE, Fujinami RS. Molecular mimicry as a mechanism of autoimmune disease. *Clin Rev Allergy Immunol.* 2012 Feb;42(1):12-11.

[24] Oldstone MB. Molecular mimicry and immune-mediated diseases. *FASEB J.* 1998 Oct;12(13):1255-65.

[25] Stevens Q, Seibly J, Chen Y, et al. Reactivation of dormant lumbar methicillin-resistant Staphylococcus aureus osteomyelitis after 12 years. *J Clin Neruosci.* 2007 jun;14(6):585-89.

[26] Castellani F, Ghidini V, Tafi MC, et al. Fate of pathogenic bacteria in microcosms mimicking human body sites. *Microb Ecol.* 2013 jul;66(1):224-31.

[27] Berthelot JM, de la Cochetiere MF, Potel G, et al. Evidence supporting a role of dormant bacteria in pathogenesis of spondyloarthritis. *Joint Bone Spine.* 2013 Mar;80(2):135-40.

[28] Berthelot JM, Glenmarec J, Guillot, et al. New pathogenic hypotheses for spondyloarthropathies. *Joint Bone Spine.* 2002 Mar;69(2):114-22.

[29] Bessome F. Non-steroidal anti-inflammatory drugs: What is the actual risk of liver damage? *World J Gasterol.* 2010 Dec 7;16(45):5851-61.

[30] Ejaz P, Bhojani K, Joshi VR. NSAIDs and kidney. *J Assoc Physicians India.* 2004 Aug;52:632-40.

[31] Gooch K, Culleton B, Manns B, et al. NSAID use and progression of chronic kidney disease. *Am J Med.* 2007 Mar;120(3):280.

[32] Bavry AA, Thomas F, Allison M, et al. Nonsteroidal anti-inflammatory drugs and cardiovascular outcomes in women: results from the women's health initiative. *Circ Cardiovasc Qual Outcomes.* 2014 Jul;7(4):603-10.

[33] Bower WA, Johns M, Margolis HS< et al. Population-based surveillance for acute liver failure. *Am J Gastroenterol.* 2007;102:2459-63.

[34] Tanne J. Paracetamol causes most liver failure in UK and US. *BMJ.* 2006 Mar;332(7542):628.

[35] American Chemical Society. The precise reason for health benefits of dark chocolate: mystery solved. Accessed August 29, 2014 from
http://www.acs.org/content/acs/en/pressroom/newsreleases/2

014/march/the-precise-reason-for-the-health-benefits-of-dark-chocolate-mystery-solved.html.

[36] di Giuseppe R, Castelnuovo A, Centritto F, et al. Regular consumption of dark chocolate is associated with low serum concentrations of C-reactive protein in a healthy Italian population. *J Nutr.* 2008 Oct;138(10):1939-45.

[37] Arita M, Bianchini F, Aliberti J, et al. Stereochemical assignment, antiinflammatory properties and receptor for the omega-3 lipid mediator resolvin E1. *JEM.* 2008 Mar;201(5):713-22.

[38] Serhan C, Resolvins and protectins: novel lipid mediators in anti-inflammation and resolution. *Scandinavian J Food Nutr.* 2006;50(52):68-78.

[39] Kohli P, Levy B. Resolvins and protectins: mediating solutions to inflammation. *Br J Pharmacol.* 2009 Oct;158(4):960-971.

[40] Grzanna R, Lindmak L, Frondoza CG. Ginger—an herbal medicinal product with broad anti-inflammatory actions. *J Med Food.* 2005 Summer;8(2):125-32.

[41] Rao C. Regulation of COX and LOX by curcumin. *Adv Exp Med Biol.* 2007;595:213-26.

[42] Guo JY, Huo HR, Zhao BS, et al. Cinnamaldehyde reduces IL-1β-induced cyclooxygenase-2 activity in rat cerebral microvascular endothelial cells. *Eur J Pharmacol.* 2006 May;537(1-3):174-80.

[43] Takenaga M, Hirai A, Terano T, et al. In vitro effect of cinnamic aldehyde, a main component of Cinnamoni Cortex, on human platelet aggregation and arachidonic acid metabolism. *J Pharmacobiodyn.* 1987 May;10(5):201-08.

[44] Shin JH, Ryu JH, Kang MJ, et al. Short-term heating reduces the anti-inflammatory effects of raw garlic extracts on the LPS-induced production of NO and pro-inflammatory cytokines by downregulating allicin activity in RAW 264.7 macrophages. *Food Chem Toxicol.* 2013 Aug;58:545-51.

[45] Belisle SE, Leka LS, Dallal GE, et al. Cytokine response to vitamin E supplementation is dependent on pre-supplementation cytokine levels. *Biofactors.* 2008;33(3):191-200.

[46] Salas-Salvado J, Casas-Argustench P, Murphy MM, et al. The effect of nuts on inflammation. *Asia Pac J Clin Nutr.* 2008;17 Suppl 1:333-36.

[47] Smith AB 3rd, Sperry JB, Han Q. Syhteses of (-)-oleocanthal, a natural NSAID found in extra virgin olive oil, the (1)-deacetoxy-oleuropein aglyconc, and related analogues. *J Org Chem.* 2007 Aug 31;72(18):6891-6900.

[48] Beauchamp GK, Keast RS, Morel D, et al. Phytochemistry: Ibuprofen-like activity in extra-virgin olive oil. *Nature.* 2005 Sep 1;437(7055):45-46.

[49] Joseph SV, Edirisinghe I, Burton-Freeman BM. Berried: Anti-inflammatory effects in humans. *J Agric Food Chem.* 2014 Mar 17. [Epub ahead of print]

[50] Wang LS, Stoner G. Anthocyanins and their role in cancer prevention. *Nat Prod.* 208 Oct;269(2):281-90.

[51] Schumacher HR, Pullman-Mooar S, Gupta SR, et al. Randomized double-blind crossover study of the efficacy of a tart cherry juice blend in treatment of osteoarthritis (OA) of the knee. *Osteoarthritis Cartilage.* 2013 Aug;21(8):1035-41.

[52] Ou B, Bosak KN, Brickner PR, et al. Processed tart cherry products—comparative phytochemical content, in vitro antioxidant capacity and in vitro anti-inflammatory activity. *J Food Sci.* 2012 May;77(5):H105-12.

[53] Wang H, Nair MG, Strasburg GM, et al. Cyclooxygenase active bioflavonoids from Balaton tart cherry and their structure activity relationships. *Phytomedicine.* 2000 Mar;7(1):15-19.

[54] Connolly D, McHugh M, Padilla-Zakour O. Efficacy of a tart cherry juice blend in preventing the symptoms of muscle damage. *Br J Sports Med.* 2006;40:679-83.

[55] Tarayre JP, Lauressergues H. Advantages of a combination of proteolytic enzymes, flavonoids and ascorbic acid in comparison with non-steroidal anti-inflammatory agents. *Arzneimittelforschung.* 1977;27(6):1144-49.

[56] Nedic O, Rattan SI, Grune T, et al. Molecular effects of advanced glycation end products on cell signaling pathways, ageing and pathophysiology. *Free Radic Res.* 2013 Aug;47 Suppl 1:28-38.

[57] David LA, Maurice CF, Carmody RN, et al. Diet rapidly and reproducibly alters the human gut microbiome. *Nature.* 2014 Jan 23;505(7484):559-63.

[58] Bicer S, Reiser PJ, Ching S, et al. Induction of muscle weakness by local inflammation: an experimental animal model. *Inflamm Res.* 2009 Apr;58(4):175-83.

[59] de Punder K, Pruimboom L. The dietary intake of wheat and other cereal grains and their role in inflammation. *Nutrients.* 2013 Mar 12;5(3):771-87.

[60] Vives MJ, Esteve M, Marine M, et al. Prevalence and clinical relevance of enteropathy associated with systemic autoimmune diseases. *Dig Liver Dis.* 2012 Aug;44(8):636-42.

[61] Togrol RE, Nalbant S, Solmazgul E, et al. The significance of celiac disease antibodies in patients with ankylosing spondylitis: a case-controlled study. *J Int Med Res.* 2009 Jan-Feb;37(1):220-26.

[62] Visser J, Rozing J, Sapone A, et al. Tight junctions, intestinal permeability, and autoimmunity celiac disease and type 1 diabetes paradigms. *Ann N Y Acad Sci.* 2009 May;1165:195-205.

[63] Manukyan G, Ghazaryan K, Ktsoyan Z, et al. Elevated systemic antibodies towards commensal gut microbiota in autoinflamamtory condition. *PLoS One.* 2008 Sep 9;3(9):e3172.

[64] Antvorskov JC, Fundova P, Buschard K, et al. Dietary gluten alters the balance of pro-inflammatory and anti-inflammatory cytokines in T Cells of BALB/c mice. *Immunology.* 2013 Jan;138(1):23-33.

[65] Soares F, Matoso R, Teixeira L, et al. Gluten-free diet reduces adiposity, inflammation and insulin resistance associated with the induction of PPAR-alpha and PPAR-gamma expression. *J Nutr Biochem.* 2013 Jun;24(6):1105-11.

[66] van Dijk SJ, Feskens EJ, Bos MB, et al. A saturated fatty acid-rich diet induces an obesity-linked proinflammatory gene expression profile in adipose tissue of subjects at risk for metabolic syndrome. *Am J Clin Nutr.* 2009 Dec;90(6):1656-64.

[67] Cullberg K, Larsen J, Pedersen S, et al. Effects of LPS and dietary free fatty acids on MCP-1 in 3T3-L1 adipocytes and macrophages in vitro. *Nutr Diabetes.* 2014 Mar;4:e113.

[68] Simopoulos AP. The importance of the ratio of omega-6/omega-3 essential fatty acids. *Biomed Pharmacother.* 2002 Oct;56(8):365-79.

[69] Oliveira MC, Menezes-Garcia Z, Henriques MC, et al. Acute and sustained inflammation and metabolic dysfunction induced by high refined carbohydrate-containing diet in mice. *Obesity (Silver Spring).* 2013 Sep;21(9):E396-406.

[70] Martini G, Brandes J. Increased consumption of refined carbohydrates in patients with Crohn's disease. *Klinische Wochenshrift.* 1976 Apr;54(8):367-71.

[71] Buyken A, Flood V, Empson M, et al. Carbohydrate nutrition and inflammatory disease mortality in older adults. *Am J Clin Nutr.* 2010 Sep;92(3):634-43.

[72] Rashid T, Wilson C, Ebringer A. The link between ankylosing spondylitis, Crohn's disease, Klebsiella, and starch consumption. *Clin Devel Immunology.* 2013 Apr;2013:872632.

[73] Rashid T, Ebringer A. Gut-mediated and HLA-B27-associated arthritis: An emphasis on ankylosing spondylitis and Crohn's disease with a proposal for the use of new treatment. *Discov Med.* 2011 Sep;12(64):187-94.

[74] Ebringer A, Wilson C. The use of a low starch diet in the treatment of patients suffering from ankylosing spondylitis. *Clin Rheumatol.* 1996 Jan;15 Suppl 1:62-66.

[75] Ley S, Sun Q, Willett W, et al. Associations between red meat intake and biomarkers of inflammation and glucose metabolism in women. *Am J Clin Nutr.* 2014 Feb:075663.

[76] Collier B, Dossett LA, May AK, et al. Glucose control and the inflammatory response. *Nutr Clin Pract.* 2008 Feb;23(1):3-15.

[77] Huber R, Hedrich A, Rostock M, et al. Clinical remission of an HLA B27-positive sacroiliitis on vegan diet. *Frosch Komplementarmed Klass Naturheilkd.* 2001 Aug;8(4):228-31.

[78] U.K. National Ankylosing Spondylitis Society. Swimming. Accessed August 29, 2014 from http://nass.co.uk/exercise/exercise-for-your-as/swimming/.

[79] Emohare O, Cagan A, Polly DW Jr, et al. Opportunistic computed tomography shows a high incidence of osteoporosis in ankylosing spondylitis patients with acute vertebral fractures. *J Clin Densitom.* 2014 Aug 26. [Epub ahead of print]

[80] Ullu MA, Batman I, Dilek B, et al. Prevalence of osteoporosis and vertebral fractures and related factors in patients with ankylosing spondylitis. *Chin Med J (Engl).* 2014 Aug;127(15):2740-47.

[81] Harper DM. ACP Journal Club. Review: Yoga reduces low back pain and back-specific disability. *Ann Intern Med.* 2013 Oct 15;159(8):JC13.

[82] Holtzman S, Beggs RT. Yoga for chronic low back pain: a meta-analysis of randomized controlled trials. *Pain Res Manag.* 2013 Sep-Oct;18(5):267-72.

[83] Cramer H, Lauche R, Haller H, et al. A systematic review and meta-analysis of yoga for low back pain. *Clin J Pain.* 2013 May;29(5):450-60.

[84] Williams K, Petronis J, Smith D, et al. Effect of Iyengar yoga therapy for chronic low back pain. *Pain.* 2005 May;115(1-2):107-17.

[85] Nambi GS, Inbasekaran D, Khuman R, et al. Changes in pain intensity and health related quality of life with Iyengar yoga in nonspecific chronic low back pain: A randomized controlled study. *Ind J Yoga.* 2014 Jan;7(1):48-53.

[86] Lee M, Moon W, Kim J. Effect of yoga on pain, brain-derived neurotrophic factor, and serotonin in premenopausal women with chronic low back pain. *Evid Based Complement Alternat Med.* 2014;214:203173.

[87] Williams K, Petronis J, Smith D, et al. Effect of Iyengar yoga therapy for chronic low back pain. *Pain.* 2005 May;115(1-2):107-17.

[88] Gallinaro AL, Akagawa LL, Otuzi MH, et al. Sexual activity in ankylosing spondylitis. *Rev Bras Rheumatol.* 2012 Dec;52(6):887-91.

[89] Sariyildiz MA, Batmaz I, Inanir A, et al. The impact of ankylosing spondylitis on female sexual intercourse. *Int J Impot Res.* 2013 May;25(3):104-08.

[90] Ozkourumak E, Karkucak M, Civil F, et al. Sexual function in male patients with ankylosing spondylitis. *Int J Impot Res*. 2011 Nov-Dec;23(6):262-67.

[91] Naziroglu M, Akkus S, Celik H. Levels of lipid peroxidation and antioxidant vitamins in plasma and erythrocytes of patients with ankylosing spondylitis. *Clin Biochem*. 2011 Dec;44(17-18):1412-15.

[92] Sundstrom B, Johansson G, Kokkonen H, et al. Plasma phospholipid fatty acid content is related to disease activity in ankylosing spondylitis. *J Rheumatol*. 2012 Feb;39(2):327-33.

[93] Sales C, Oliviero F, Spinella P. Role of omega-3 polyunsaturated fatty acids in diet of patients with rheumatic diseases. *Rheumatismo*. 2008 Apr-Jun;60(2):95-101.

[94] Calder PC. Marine omega-3 fatty acids and inflammatory process: Effects, mechanisms and clinical evidence. *Biochem Biophys Acta*. 2014 Aug 20. [Epub ahead of print]

[95] Mori TA. Omega-3 fatty acids and cardiovascular disease: epidemiology and effects on cardiometabolic risk factors. *Food Funct*. 2014 Aug 20;5(9):2004-19.

[96] Sandstrom B, Stalnacke K, Hagfors L, et al. Supplementation of omega-3 fatty acids in patients with ankylosing spondylitis. *Scand J Rheumatol*. 2006 Sep-Oct;35(5):359-62.

[97] Tlaskalova-Hogenova H, Stepankova R, Kozakova H, et al. The role of gut microbiota (commensal bacteria) and the mucosal barrier in the pathogenesis of inflammatory and autoimmune diseases and cancer: contribution of gem-free and gnotobiotic animal models of human diseases. *Cell Mol Immunol*. 2011 Mar;8(2):110-20.

[98] Vaghef-Mehrabany E, Alipour B, Homayouni-Rad-A, et al. Probiotic supplementation improves inflammatory status in patients with rheumatoid arthritis. *Nutrition*. 2014 Apr;30(4):430-50.

[99] Pineda Mde L, Thjompson SF, Summers K, et al. A randomized, double-blinded, placebo-controlled pilot study of probiotics in active rheumatoid arthritis. *Med Sci Monit*. 2011 jun;17(6):CR347-54.

[100] Baharav E, Mor F, Halpern M, et al. Lactobacillus GG bacteria ameliorate arthritis in Lewis rats. *J Nutr.* 2004 Aug;134(8):1964-99.

[101] Amdekar S, Singh V, Singh R, et al. Lactobacillus casei reduces inflammatory joint damage associated with collagen-induced arthritis (CIA) by reducing the pro-inflammatory cytokines: Lactobacilus casei: COX-2 inhibitor. *J Clin Immunol.* 2011 Apr;31(2):147-54.

[102] Karimi O, Pena AS. Probiotics in arthralgia and spondyloarthropathies in patients with inflammatory bowel disease. Prospective randomized trials are necessary. *Rev Esp Enferm Dig.* 2005 Aug;97(8):570-74.

[103] Zhang F, Altorki NK, Mestre JR, et al. Curcumin inhibits cyclooxygenase-2 transcription in bile acid- and phorbol ester-treated human gastrointestinal epithelial cells. *Carcinogenesis.* 1999;20:445-51.

[104] Koeberle A, Northoff H, Werz O. Curcumin blocks prostaglandin E2 biosynthesis through direct inhibition of the microsomal prostaglandin E2 synthase-1. *Mol Cancer Ther. 2009 Aug;8(8):2348-55.*

[105] Abe Y, Hashimoto S, Horie T. Curcumin inhibition of inflammatory cytokine production by human peripheral blood monocytes and alveolar macrophages. *Pharmacol Res.* 1999 Jan;39(1):41-47.

[106] Ammon HP, Anazodo MI, Safayhi H, et al. Curcumin: a potent inhibitor of leukotriene B4 formation in rat peritoneal polymorphonuclear neutrophils (PMNL). *Planta Med.* 1992 Apr;58(2):226.

[107] Aggarwal BB, Gupta SC, Sung B. Curcumin: an orally bioavailable blocker of TNF and other pro-inflammatory biomarkers. *BR J Pharmacol.* 2013 Aug;169(8):1672-92.

[108] Gupta SC, Tyagi AK, Deshmukh-Taskar P, et al. Downregualtion of tumor necrosis factor and other proinflammatory biomarkers by polyphenols. *Arch Biochem Biophys.* 2014 Oct 1;559C:91-99.

[109] Taty Anna K, Elvy Suhana MR, Das S, et al. Anti-inflammatory effect of Curcuma longa (turmeric) on collagen-induced arthritis: an anatomicro-radiological study. *Clin Ter.* 2011;162(3):201-07.

[110] Di Pierro F, Rapacioli G, Di Maio EA, et al. Comparative evaluation of the pain-relieving properties of a lecithinized formulation of curcumin (Meriva®), nimesulide, and acetaminophen. *J Pain Res.* 2013;6:201-05.

[111] Baum L, Lam CW, Cheung SK, et al. Six-month randomized, placebo-controlled, double-blind, pilot clinical trial of curcumin in patients with Alzheimer's disease (letter). *J Clin Psychopharmacol.* 2008;28:110-13.

[112] Srivastava KC, Mustafa T. Ginger (Zingiber officinale) and rheumatic disorders. *Med Hypotheses.* 1989 May;29(1):25-28.

[113] Grzanna R, Lindmark L, Frondoza C. Ginger—An herbal medicinal product with broad anti-inflammatory actions. *J Med Food.* 2005 Jul;8(2):125-32.

[114] Srivastava KC, Mustafa T. Ginger (Zingiber officinale) in rheumatism and musculoskeletal disorders. *Med Hypotheses.* 1992 Dec;39(4):342-48.

[115] Frondoza CG, Sohrabi A, Polotsky A, et al. An in vitro screening assay for inhibitors of proinflammatory mediators in herbal extracts using human synoviocyte cultures. *In Vitro Cell Biol Anim.* 2004;40:95-101.

[116] Thomson M, Al-Quattan KK, Al-Sawan SM, et al. The use of ginger (Zingiber officinale Rosc.) as a potential anti-inflammatory and antithrombotic agent. *Prostaglandins Leukot Essent Fatty Acids.* 2002 Dec;67(6):475-78.

[117] Al-Nahaim A, Jahan R, Rahmatullah M. Zingiber officinale: A potential plant against rheumatoid arthritis. *Arthritis.* 2014:2014:159089.

[118] Sritoomma N, Moyle W, Cooke M, et al. The effectiveness of Swedish massage with aromatic ginger oil in treating chronic low back pain in older adults: a randomized controlled trial. *Complement Ther Med.* 2014 Feb;22(1):26-33.

[119] Murav'ev IuV, Venikova MS, Pleskovskaia GN, et al. Effect of dimethyl sulfoxide and dimethyl sulfone on a destructive process in the joints of mice with spontaneous arthritis. *Patol Fiziol Eksp Ter.* 1991 May-Apr;(2):37-39.

[120] Brien S, Prescott P, Lewith G. Meta-analysis of the related nutritional supplements dimethyl sulfoxide and methylsulfonylmethane in the treatment of osteoarthritis of

the knee. *Evid Based Complement Alternat Med.* 2011;2011:528403.

[121] Usha PR, Naidu MUR, Randomised double-blind, parallel, placebo-controlled study of oral glucosamine, methylsulfonylmethane and their combination in osteoarthritis. *Clin Drug Invest.* 2004 Jun;24(6):353-63.

[122] Floss BL, Maxwell TW, Deng Y. Chondroprotective supplementation promotes the mechanical properties of injectable scaffold for human nucleus pulposus tissue engineering. *J Mech Behav Biomed Mater.* 2014 Jan;29:56-67.

[123] Blitterswijk W, van de Nes J, Wuisman P. Glucosamine and chondroitin sulfate supplementation to treat symptomatic disc degeneration: Biochemical rationale and case report. *BMC Comp Altern Med.* 2003 Jun;10(3):2.

[124] Morton JI, Siegel BV. Effects of oral dimethyl sulfoxide and dimethyl sulfone on murine autoimmune lymphoproliferative disease. *Proc Soc Exp Biol Med.* 1986 Nov;183(2):227-30.

[125] Rees WD, Rhodes J, Wright JE, et al. Effect of deglycyrrhizinated liquorice on gastric mucosal damage by aspirin. *Scand J Gastroenterol.* 1979;14(5):605-07.

[126] Das SK, Das V, Gulati AK, et al. Deglycyrrhizinated liquorice in aphthous ulcers. *J Assoc Physicians India.* 1989 Oct;37(10):647.

[127] Methlie P, Husebye EE, Hustad S, et al. Grapefruit juice and licorice increase cortisol availability in patients with Addison's disease. *Eur J Endocrinol.* 2011 Nov;165(5):761-69.

[128] Ammon HP. Boswellic acids in chronic inflammatory diseases. *Planta Med.* 2006 Oct;72(12):1100-16.

[129] Ammon HP. Boswellic acids (components of frankincense) as active principle in treatment of chronic inflammatory diseases. *Wien Med Wochenschr.* 2002;152(15-16):373-78.

[130] Bishnoi M, Patil CS, Kumar A, et al. Protective effects of nimesulide (COX inhibitor), AKBA (5-LOX inhibitor), and their combination in aging-associated abnormalities in mice. *Methods Find Exp Clin Pharmacol.* 2005 Sep;27(7):465-70.

[131] Ammon HP. Modulation of the immune system by Boswellia serrata extracts and boswellic acids. *Phytomedicine.* 2010 Sep;17(11):862-67.
[132] Wildfeuer A, Neu IS, Safayhi H, et al. Effects of boswellic acids extracted from a herbal medicine on the biosynthesis of leukotrienes and the course of experimental autoimmune encephalomyelitis. *Arzneimittelforschung.* 1998;48:668-74.
[133] Sturner K, Verse N, Yousef S, et al. Boswellic acids reduce TH17 differentiation via blockade of IL-1β-Mediated IRAK1 signaling. *Eur J Immunol.* 2014 Apr;44(4):120-12.
[134] Pham C, Neutropjil serine proteases: specific regulators of inflammation. *Nature Rev Immunology.* 2006 Jul;5:541-50.
[135] Vergnolle N, Walalce J, Bunnett N, et al. Protease-activated receptors in inflammation, neuronal signaling and pain. *Trends Pharmacol Sci.* 2001 Mar;22(3):146-52.
[136] Selim SA, Adam ME, Hassan SM, et al. Chemical composition, antimicrobial and antibiofilm activity of the essential oil and methanol extract of the Mediterranean cypress (Cupressus sempervirens L.). *BMC Complement Altern Med.* 2014 Jun 2;14:179.
[137] Warnke PH, Lott AJ, Sherry E, et al. The ongoing battle against multi-resistant strains: in-vitro inhibition of hospital-acquired MRSA, VRE, Pseudomonas, ESBL E. coli and Klebsiella species in the presence of plant-derived antiseptic oils. *J Craniomaxillofac Surg.* 2013 Jun;41(5):321-26.
[138] Orhan IE, Ozcelik B, Kan Y, et al. Inhibitory effects of various essential oils and individual components against extended-spectrum beta-lactamase (ESBL) produced by Klebsiella pneumonia and their chemical compositions. *J Food Sci.* 2001 Oct;76(8):M538-46.
[139] Thosar N, Basak S, Bahadure RN, et al. Antimicrobial efficacy of five essential oils against oral pathogens: An in vitro study. *Eur J Dent.* 2013 Sep;7(Suppl 1):S71-77.
[140] SienkieWicz M, Lysakowska M, Pastuszka M, et al. The potential use of basil and rosemary essential oils as effective antibacterial agents. *Molecules.* 2013 Aug 5;18(8):9334-51.
[141] Santoyo S, Cavero S, Jaime L, et al. Supercritical carbon dioxide extraction of compounds with antimicrobial activity

from Origanum vulgare L.: determination of optimal extraction parameters. *J Food Prot.* 2006 Feb;69(2):369-75.

[142] Malik T, Singh P, Pant S, et al. Potentiation of antimicrobial activity of ciprofloxacin by Pelargonium essential oil against selected uropathogens. *Phytother Res.* 211 Aug;25(8):1225-28.

[143] Aggarwai K, Ateeque A, Kumar T, et al. Antimicrobial activity spectra of Pelargonium graveolens L. and Cymbopogon winterianus Jowitt oil constituents and acyl derivatives. *J Med Aromatic Plant Sci.* 2000;22(1B):544-48.

[144] Bachir RG, Benali M. Antibacterial activity of the essential oils from the leaves of Eucalyptus globulus against Escherichia coli and Staphylococcus aureus. *Asian Pac J Biomed.* 2012 Sep;2(9):739-42.

[145] Fabio A, Cermelli C, Fabio G, et al. Screening of the antimicrobial effects of a variety of essential oils on microorganisms responsible for respiratory infections. *Phytother Res.* 2007 Apr;21(4):374-77.

[146] Hammer KA, Carson CF, Riley TV. Antimicrobial activity of essential oils and other plant extracts. *J Appl Microbiol.* 1999 Jun;86(6):985-90.

[147] Chaudhary SC, Siddiqui MS, Athar M, et al. D-limonene modulates inflammation, oxidative stress and Ras-ERK pathway to inhibit murine skin tumorigenesis. *Hum Exp Toxicol.* 2012 Aug;31(8):798-811.

[148] Iannitti T, Morales-Medina JC, Bellavite P, et al. Effectiveness and safety of Arnica montana in post-surgical setting, pain and inflammation. 2014 Sep 17. [Epub ahead of print]

[149] Burks TF, Buck SH, Miller MS. Mechanisms of depletion of substance P by capsaicin. *Fed Proc.* 1985 Jun;44(9):2531-34

[150] Anand P, Bley K. Topical capsaicin for pain management: therapeutic potential and mechanisms of action of the new high-concentration capsaicin 8% patch. *Br J Anaesth.* 2011 Oct;107(4):490-502.

[151] Uhl RL, Roberts TT, Papaliodis, et al. Management of chronic musculoskeletal pain. *J Am Acad Orthop Surg.* 2014 Feb;22(2):101-10.

[152] Singh BB, Mishra L, Aquilina N, Kohlbeck F. Usefulness of guggl (Commiphora mukul) for osteoarthritis of the knee: An experimental case study. *Altern Ter Health Med.* 2001 Mar;7(2);120, 112-14.

[153] Samarasinghe RM, Kanwar RK, Kumar K, et al. Antiarthritic and chondroprotective activity of Lakshadi Guggul in novel alginate-enclosed chitosan calcium phosphate nanocarriers. *Nonomedicine (Lond).* 2014 May;9(6):819-37.

[154] Gayathri B, Manjula N, Vinaykumar KS, et al. Pure compound from Boswellia serrata extract exhibits antiinflammatory property in human PBMCs and mouse macrophages through inhibition of TNFalpha, IL-1beta, NO and MAP kinases. *Int Immunopharmacol.* 2007 Apr;7(4):473-82.

[155] Gebhard C, Stampfli SF, Gebhard CE, et al. Guggulsterone, an anti-inflammatory phytosterols, inhibits tissue factor and arterial thrombosis. *Basic Res Cardiol.* 2009 May;14(3):285-94.

[156] Song JJ, Kwon SK, Cho CG, et al. Guggulsterone suppresses LPS induced inflammation of human middle ear epithelial cells (HMEEC). *Int J Pediatr Otorhinolaryngol.* 2010 Dec;74(12):1384-7.

[157] Deng R. Therapeutic effects of guggul and its constituent guggulsterone: Cardiovascular benefits. *Card Drug Rev.* 2007 Winer;25(4):375-90.

[158] Zhao S, Duffield SJ, Moots RJ, et al. Systematic review of association between vitamin D levels and susceptibility and disease activity of ankylosing spondylitis. *Rheumatology (Oxford).* 2014 Sep;53(9):1595-1603.

[159] Durmus B, Altay Z, Baysal O, et al. Does vitamin D affect disease severity in patients with ankylosing spondylitis. *Clin Med J (Engl).* 2012 Jul;125(14):2511-15.

[160] Zhang Y, Leung D, Richers B, et al. Vitamin D inhibits monocyte/macrophage proinflammatory cytokine production by targeting MAPK phosphatase-1. *J Immunology.* 2012 Mar;188(5):2127-35.

[161] Waterhouse JC, Perez TH, Albert PJ. Reversing bacteria-induced vitamin D receptor dysfunction is key to

autoimmune disease. *Ann N Y Acad Sci.* 2009 Sep;1173:757-65.

[162] Obermayer-Pietsch BM, Lange U, Tauber G, et al. Vitamin D receptor initiation codon polymorphism, bone density and inflammatory activity of patients with ankylosing spondylitis. *Osteoporosis Int.* 2003 Dec;14(12):995-1000.

[163] Schauber J, Gallo R. The vitamin D pathway: a new target for control of the skin's immune response? *Exp Dematol.* 2008 Aug;17(8):633-39.

[164] Ben-Zvi I, Aranow C, Mackay M, et al. The impact of vitamin D on dendritic cell function in patients with systemic lupus erythematosus. *PLoS One.* 2010 Feb 16;5(2):e9193.

[165] Park, JS, Chyun JH, Kim YK, et al. Astaxanthin decreased oxidative stress and inflammation and enhanced immune response in humans. *Nutr Metab (Lond).* 2010 Mar 5;7:18.

[166] Spiller G, Dewell A, Chaves S, et al. Effect of daily use natural astaxanthin on C-reactive protein. Accessed September 3, 2014 from http://www.astaxanthin.org/pdfs/batl43.pdf.

[167] Andersen LP, Holck S, Kupcinskas L, et al. Gastric inflammatory markers and interleukins in patients with functional dyspepsia treated with astaxanthin. *FEMS Immunol Med Microbiol.* 2007;50(2):244-48.

[168] Ohgami K, Shiratori K, Kotake S, et al. Effects of astaxanthin on lipopolysaccharide-induced inflammation in vitro and in vivo. *Invest Opthamol.* 2003 Jun'44(6):2694-2701.

[169] Guerin M, Huntley M, Olaizola M. Haematococcus astaxanthin: applications for human health and nutrition. *Trends Biotech.* 2003 May;21(5):210-16.

[170] Kurashige M, Okimasu E, Inoue M, et al. Inhibition of oxidative injury of biological membranes by astaxanthin. *Physiol Chem Phys & Med.* 1990,22.27-38.

[171] Smith VH. Vitamin C deficiency is an under-diagnosed contributor to degenerative disc disease in the elderly. *Med Hypotheses.* 2010 Apr;74(4):695-97.

[172] Wintergerst ES, Maggini S, Hornig DH. Immune-enhancing role of vitamin C and zinc and effect on clinical conditions. *Ann Nutr Metab.* 2006;50(2):85-94.

[173] Imai S. The NAD world: a new systematic regulatory network for metabolism and aging--Sirt1, systematic NAD biosynthesis, and their importance.

[174] Chi Y, Sauve AA. Nicotinamide ribose, a trace nutrient in foods, is a vitamin B3 with effects on energy metabolism and neuroprotection. *Curr Opin Clin Nutr Metab Care.* 2013 nov;16(6):657-61.

[175] Tullius SG, Biefer HRC, Li S, et al. NAD^+ protects against EAE by regulating $CD4^+$ T-cell differentiation. *Nature Communications.* 2014 Oct 7;5101(5):1-17.

[176] Gomes AP, Price NL, Ling JY, et al. Declining NAD^+ induces a pseudohypoxic state disrupting nuclear-mitochondrial communication during aging. *Cell.* 2013 Dec;155(7):1624-38.

[177] Visalli N, Cavallo MG, Signore A, et al. A multi-centre randomized trial of two different doses of nicotinamide in patients with recent-onset type 1 diabetes (The IMDIAB VI) *Diabetes Metab Res Rev.* 1999;15:181-85.

[178] Chahine L, Sempson N, Wagoner C. The effect of sodium lauryl sulfate on recurrent aphthous ulcers: a clinical study. *Compend Contin Educ Dent.* 1997 Dec;18(12):1238-40.

[179] Burgess J, van der Ven P, Martin M, et al. Review of over-the-counter treatments for the aphthous ulceration and results from use of a dissolving oral patch containing glycyrrhiza complex herbal patch. *J Cont Dent Pract.* 2008 Mar;9(3):1-15.

[180] Pedersen A, Hougen HP, Klausen B, et al. LongoVital in the prevention of recurrent aphthous ulcers. *J Oral Pathol Med.* 1990;19:371-75.

[181] Rudwaleit M, Baeten D. Ankylosing spondylitis and bowel disease. *Best Pract Res Clin Rheumatol.* 2006 Jun;20(3):451-71.

[182] Felder J, Korelitz B, Rajapaske R, et al. Effects of nonsteroidal antiinflammatory drugs on inflammatory bowel disease: a case-control study. *Am J Gastroenterology.* 2000 Aug;95(8):1949-54.

[183] Khanna R, MacDonald JK, Levesque BG. Peppermint oil for the treatment of irritable bowel syndrome: a systematic review and meta-analysis. *J Clin Gastroenterol.* 2014 Jul;48(6):505-12.

[184] Langmead L, Dawson C, Hawkins C, et al. Antioxidant effects of herbal therapies used by patients with inflammatory bowel disease: an in vitro study. *Alimentary Pharmacol Ther.* 2002 Feb;16(2):197-205.

[185] Feng D, Xu W, Chen G, et al. Influence of glutamine on intestinal inflammatory response, mucosa structure alterations and apoptosis following traumatic brain injury in rats. *J Int Med Res.* 2007 Sep-Oct;35(5):644-56.

[186] Langmead L, Feakins RM, Goldsthorpe S, et al. Randomized, double-blind, placebo-controlled trial of oral aloe vera gel for active ulcerative colitis. *Ailment Pharmacol Ther.* 2004 Apr 1;19(7):739-47.

[187] Suzuki T, Hara H. Quercetin enhances intestinal barrier function through the assembly of zonnula occludens-2, occluding, and claudin-1 and the expression of claudin-4 in caco-2 cells. *J Nutr.* 2009 May;139(5):965-74.

[188] Amasheh M, Schlichter S, Amasheh S, et al. Quercetin enhances epithelial barrier function and increases claudin-4 expression in caco-2 cells. *J Nutr.* 2008 Jun;138(6):1067-73.

[189] Noda S, Tanabe S, Suzuki T. Naringenin enhances intestinal barrier function through the expression and cytoskeletal association of tight junction proteins in Caco-2 cells. *Mol Nutr Food Res.* 2013 Nov;57(11):2019-28.

[190] Iraha A, Chinen H, Hokama A, et al. Fucoidan enhances intestinal barrier function by upregulating the expression of claudin-1. *World Gastroenterol.* 2013 Sep 7;19(33):5500-07.

[191] Wang B, Wu G, Zhou Z, et al. Glutamine and intestinal barrier function. *Amino Acids.* 2014 Jun 26. [Epub ahead of print]

[192] Zuhl MN, Lanphere KR, Kravitz L, et al. Effects of oral glutamine supplementation on exercise-induced gastrointestinal permeability and tight junction protein expression. *J Appl Physiol (1985).* 2014 Jan 15;116(2):183-91.

[193] Lautermann D, Braun J. Ankylosing spondylitis — cardiac manifestations. *Clin Exp Rheumatology.* 2002;20(Suppl 28):S11-15.

[194] Roman M, Salmon J. Cardiovascular involvement in general medical conditions. *Circulation.* 2007;116:2346-55.

[195] Lui NL, Thumboo J, Inman R. Cardiomyopathy in ankylosing spondylitis. 2011 Apr;63(4):564-69.

[196] Chen Y, Chung HY, Zhao CT, et al. Left ventricular myocardial dysfunction and premature atherosclerosis in patients with axial spondyloarthritis. *Rheumatology (Oxford).* 2014 Aug 29. [Epub ahead of print]

[197] Dai YL, Luk TH, Yiu KH, et al. Reversal of mitochondrial dysfunction by coenzyme Q10 supplement improves endothelial function in patients with ischaemic left ventricular systolic dysfunction: a randomized controlled trial. *Atherosclerosis.* 2011 Jun;216(2):395-401.

[198] Kishimoto C, Tomioka N, Nakayama Y, et al. Anti-oxidant effects of coenzyme Q10 on experimental viral myocarditis in mice. *J Cardiovasc Pharmacol.* 2003 Nov;42(5):588-92.

[199] Mollet J, Giurgea I, Schlemmer D, et al. Prenyldiphosphate synthase, subunit 1 (PDSS1) and OH-benzoate polyprenyltransferase (COQ2) mutations in ubiquinone deficiency and oxidative phosphorylation disorders. *J Clin Invest.* 2007 Mar;117(3):765-72.

[200] Gao L, Mao Q, Cao J, et al. Effects of coenzyme Q10 on vascular endothelial function in humans: a meta-analysis of randomized controlled trials. *Atherosclerosis.* 2012 Apr;221(2):311-16.

[201] Sacher HL, Sacher ML, Landau SW, et al. The clinical and hemodynamic effects of coenzyme Q10 in congestive cardiomyopathy. *Am J Ther.* 1997 Feb-Mar;4(2-3):66-72.

[202] Usharani P, Fatima N, Muralidhar. Effects of Phyllanthus embillica extract on endothelial dysfunction and biomarkers of oxidative stress in patients with type 2 diabetes mellitus: a randomized, double-blind, controlled study. *Diabetes Metab Syndr Obes.* 2013 Jul 26;6:275-84.

[203] Rajak S, Banerjee Sk, Sood S, et al. Embilica officinalis causes myocardial adaptation and protects against oxidative stress in ischemic-reperfusion injury in rats. *Phytother Res.* 2004 Jan;18(1):54-60.

[204] Wang YF, Wang Xy, Ren Z, et al. Phyllaemblicin B inhibits Coxsackie virus B3 induced apoptosis and myocarditis. *Antiviral Res.* 2009 Nov;84(2):150-58.

[205] Ojha S, Golechha M, Kumari S, et al. Protective effect of Embilica officinalis (amla) on isoproterenol-induced cardiotoxicity in rats. *Toxicol Ind Health.* 2012 Jun;28(5):399-411.

[206] Wattanapitayakul SK, Chularojmontri L, Herunsalee A, et al. Screening of antioxidants from medicinal plants for cardioprotective effect against doxorubicin toxicity. *Basic Clin Pharmacol Toxicol.* 2005 Jan;96(1):80-87.

[207] Mitre R, Etienne M, Martinais S, et al. Humoral defence improvement and haematopoiesis in sows and offspring by oral supply of shark-liver oil to mothers during gestation and lactation. *Br J Nutr.* 2005 Nov;94(5):753-62.

[208] Pogozheva AV, Derbeneva SA, Anykina NV, et al. The clinical and experimental research of metabolic effects of shark liver oil. *Vopr Pitan.* 2007;76(6):28-32.

[209] Li SD, Su YD, Li M, et al. Hemin-induced hemolysis in erythrocytes: effects of ascorbic acid and glutathione. *Acta Biochim Biophys Sin (Shanghai).* 2006 Jan;38(1):63-69.

[210] Choi YD, Park CW, Jang J, et al. Effects of Korean ginseng-berry extract on sexual function in men with erectile dysfunction: a multicenter, placebo-controlled, double-blind clinical study. *Int J Impor Res.* 2013 Mar-Apr;25(2):45-50.

[211] Kim TH, Jeon SH, Hahn EJ, et al. Effects of tissue-cultured mountain ginseng (Panax ginseng CA Meyer) extract on male patients with erectile dysfunction. *Asian J Androl.* 2009 May;11(3):356-61.

[212] Stanislavov R, Nikolova V. Treatment of erectile dysfunction with pycnogenol and L-arginine. *J Sex Marital Ther.* 2003 May-Jun;29(3):207-13.

[213] Chen J, Wollman Y, Chernichovsky T, et al. Effect of oral administration of high-dose nitric oxide donor L-arginine in men with organic erectile dysfunction: results of a double-blind, randomized, placebo-controlled study. *BJU Int.* 1999;83:269-73.

[214] Kanathur N, Lee-Chiong T. Pulmonary manifestations of ankylosing spondylitis. *Clin Chest Med.* 2010 Sep;31(3):547-54.

[215] Hasiloglu Z, Havan N, Rezvani A, et al. Lung parenchymal changes in patients with ankylosing spondylitis. *World J Radiol.* 2012 May;4(5):215-19.

[216] Mangprayool T, Kupittayanant S, Chudaprongse N. Participation of citral in the bronchodilatory effect of ginger oil and possible mechanisms of action. *Fitoterapia.* 2013 Sep;89:68-73.

[217] Janbaz KH, Nisa M, Saqib F, et al. Bronchodilator, vasodilator and spasmolytic activities of methanolic extract of Myrtus communis L. *J Phys Pharmacol.* 2003 Aug;64(4):479-84.

[218] Rao BS, Shanbhoge R, Rao BN, et al. Preventive efficacy of hydroalcoholic extract of Cymbopogon citratus against radiation-induced DNA damage on V79 cells and free radical scavenging ability against radicals generated in vitro. *Hum Exp Toxicol.* 2009 Apr;28(4):195-202.

[219] Shah G, Shri R, Panchal V, et al. Scientific basis for the therapeutic use of Cymbopogon citratus, stapf (Lemon grass). *J Adv Pharm Technol Res.* 2011 Jan;2(1):3-8.

[220] Nascimento NR, Refosco RM, Vasconcelos ES, et al. 1,8-Cineole induces relaxation in rat and guinea-pig airway smooth muscle. *J Pharm Pharmacol.* 2009 Mar;61(3):361-66.

[221] Zhao W, Wang Y, Tang FD, et al. The expression of TLR4 in rat acute lung injury induced by lipopolysaccharide and the influence of Eucalyptus globulus oil. *Zhongguo Zhong Yao Za Zhi.* 2006 Feb;31(4):319-22.

[222] Bhagat M, Sharma V, Saxena AK. Anti-proliferative effect of leaf extracts of Eucalyptus citridora against human cancer cells in vitro and in vivo. *Indian J Biochem Biophys.* 2012 Dec;49(6):451-57.

[223] Zhu JS, Halpern GM, Jones K. The scientific rediscovery of an ancient Chinese herbal medicine: Cordyceps sinensis: part 1. *J Altern Complement Med.* 1998;4:289-303.

[224] Zhu JS, Halpern GM, Jones K. The scientific rediscovery of an ancient Chinese herbal medicine: Cordyceps sinensis: part 2. *J Altern Complement Med.* 1998;4:429-57.

[225] Yan W, Li T, Lao J, et al. Anti-fatigue property of Cordyceps guangdongensis and the underlying mechanisms. *Pharm Biol.* 213 May;51(5):614-20.

[226] Kumar R, Negi PS, Singh B, et al. Cordyceps sinensis promotes exercise endurance capacity of rats by activating

skeletal muscle metabolic regulators. *J Ethnopharmacol.* 2011 Jun 14;136(1):260-66.

[227] Chen S, Li Z, Krochmal R, et al. Effect of Cs-4 (Cordyceps sinensis) on exercise performance in healthy older subjects: a double-blind, placebo-controlled trial. *J Altern Complement Med.* 2010 May;16(5):585-90.

[228] Zhang C, Yang X, Xu L. Immunomodulatory action of the total saponin of Gynostemma pentaphylla. *Zhong XI Yi Jie He Za Zhi.* 1990 Feb;10(2):96-98, 69-70.

[229] Jiang Y, Yang M, Wu H, et al. The relationship between disease activity measured by the BASDAI and psychological status, stressful life events, and sleep quality in ankylosing spondylitis. *Clin Rhematol.* 2014 Jun 20. [Epub ahead of print]

[230] Li Y, Zhang S, Zhu J, et al. Sleep disturbances are associated with increased pain, disease activity, depression, and anxiety in ankylosing spondylitis. *Arthritis Res Ther.* 2012 Oct 11;14(5):R215.

[231] Samborski W, Sobieska M, Mackiewicz T, et al. Can thermal therapy of ankylosing spondylitis induce an activation of the disease? *Z Rheumatol.* 1992 May-Jun;51(3):127-31.

[232] Banfi G, Lombardi G, Colombini A, et al. Whole-body cryotherapy in athletes. *Sports Med.* 2010 Jun 1;40(6):509-17.

[233] Lange U, Uhlemann C, Muller-Ladner U. Serial whole-body cryotherapy in the criostream for inflammatory rheumatic diseases. A pilot study. *Med Klin (Munich).* 2008 Jun 15;103(6):383-88.

[234] Metzger D, Zwingmann C, Protz W, et al. Whole-body cryotherapy in rehabilitation of patients with rheumatoid diseases--pilot study. Die *Rehabilitation.* 2000 Apr;39(2):93-100.

[235] Stanek A, Sierorl A, Cieslar G, et al. The impact of whole-body cryotherapy on parameters of spinal mobility in patients with ankylosing spondylitis. *Ortop Traumatic Rehabili.* 2005 Oct 30;7(5):549-54.

[236] Martindale J, Smith J, Sutton J, et al. Disease and psychological status in ankylosing spondylitis. *Rheumatology.* 2006;45(10):1288-93.

[237] Ortancil O, Konuk N, May H, et al. Psychological status and patient-assessed health instruments in ankylosing spondylitis. J Clin Rheumatol. 2010 Oct;16(7):313-16.

[238] Hakkou J, Rostrom S, Aissaoui N, et al. Psychological status in Moroccan patients with ankylosing spondylitis and its relationship with disease parameters and quality of life. *J Clin Rheumatol.* 2011 Dec;17(8):424-28.

[239] Baysal O, Durmus B, Ersoy Y, et al. Relationship between psychological status and disease activity and quality of life in ankylosing spondylitis. *Rheumatol Int.* 2011 Jun;31(6):795-800.

[240] Stinger J, Swindell R, Dennis M. Massage in patients undergoing intensive chemotherapy reduces serum cortisol and prolactin. *Psycho-Oncology.* 2008 oct;17(10):1024-31.

[241] Mizreal F, Keshtgar S, Kaviani M, et al. The effect of lavender essence smelling during labor on cortisol and serotonin plasma levels and anxiety reduction in nulliparous women. *J Kerman Univ Med Sci Health Serv.* 2009 Summer;16(3).

Made in the USA
Middletown, DE
09 August 2023